ACLS
STUDY CARDS

ACLS
STUDY CARDS

Third Edition

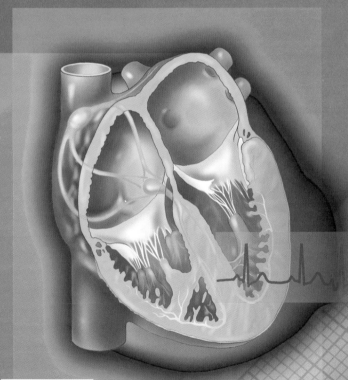

Barbara Aehlert, RN, BSPA

Southwest EMS Education, Inc.
Phoenix, Arizona/Pursley, Texas

MOSBY JEMS

ELSEVIER

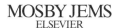

MOSBY JEMS
ELSEVIER

11830 Westline Industrial Drive
St. Louis, Missouri 63146

ACLS STUDY CARDS
ISBN: 978-0-323-05810-0
Copyright © 2009, 2004, 2001 by Mosby, Inc., an affiliate of Elsevier Inc.

Notice

Knowledge and best practice in this field are constantly changing. As new research and experience broaden our knowledge, changes in practice, treatment and drug therapy may become necessary or appropriate. Readers are advised to check the most current information provided (i) on procedures featured or (ii) by the manufacturer of each product to be administered, to verify the recommended dose or formula, the method and duration of administration, and contraindications. It is the responsibility of the practitioner, relying on their own experience and knowledge of the patient, to make diagnoses, to determine dosages and the best treatment for each individual patient, and to take all appropriate safety precautions. To the fullest extent of the law, neither the Publisher nor the Editors assumes any liability for any injury and/or damage to persons or property arising out of or related to any use of the material contained in this book.

The Publisher

Executive Editor: Linda Honeycutt
Associate Developmental Editor: Mary Jo Adams
Publishing Services Manager: Julie Eddy
Senior Project Manager: Celeste Clingan
Design Direction: Amy Buxton

Printed in Canada

Last digit is the print number: 9 8 7 6 5 4 3 2 1

NOTE TO THE READER

- These ACLS cards are designed to assist you in learning the material presented in the ACLS Provider (Student) Course. The cards are presented in the following categories:

  - ABCDs of Emergency Cardiac Care
  - Airway Management
  - Rhythm Recognition
  - Electrical Therapy
  - Vascular Access and Medications
  - Acute Coronary Syndromes
  - Stroke and Special Resuscitation Situations
  - Putting it all Together

- The cards are presented in random order within each category.

- Determination of heart rate on these cards will require calculation using the large box or small box method. Use of an ECG ruler will result in **inaccurate** results because the rhythm strips have been reduced in size.

ABOUT THE AUTHOR

Barbara Aehlert RN, BSPA, is the President of Southwest EMS Education, Inc., Phoenix, Arizona and Pursley, Texas. She has been a registered nurse for more than 30 years, with clinical experience in medical/surgical and critical care nursing and, for the past 21 years, in prehospital education. Barbara is an active CPR, First Aid, ACLS, and PALS instructor. She is the Director of Field Training for Southwest Ambulance in Mesa, Arizona, and an active member of the Pursley, Texas, Volunteer Fire Department.

CONTENTS

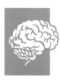

ABCDs of Emergency Cardiac Care

What is sudden cardiac death?

ABCDs of Emergency Cardiac Care

ABCDs of Emergency Cardiac Care

Explain the term "cardiovascular disorders."

ABCDs of Emergency Cardiac Care

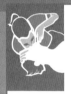

Name four cardiac arrest rhythms.

ABCDs of Emergency Cardiac Care

What are risk factors?

ABCDs of Emergency Cardiac Care

What is "public access defibrillation"?

ABCDs of Emergency Cardiac Care

Name four nonmodifiable risk factors for coronary artery disease.

ABCDs of Emergency Cardiac Care

Name the four links in the chain of survival.

ABCDs of Emergency Cardiac Care

ABCDs of Emergency Cardiac Care

Sudden cardiac death is an unexpected death of cardiac etiology occurring either immediately or within 1 hour of onset of symptoms.

ABCDs of Emergency Cardiac Care

- Pulseless ventricular tachycardia
- Ventricular fibrillation
- Asystole
- Pulseless electrical activity

ABCDs of Emergency Cardiac Care

Cardiovascular disorders are a collection of diseases and conditions that involve the heart (cardio) and blood vessels (vascular).

ABCDs of Emergency Cardiac Care

"Public access defibrillation" refers to defibrillation performed at the scene by laypersons.

ABCDs of Emergency Cardiac Care

Risk factors are traits and lifestyle habits that may increase a person's chance of developing a disease. More than 300 risk factors have been associated with coronary heart disease and stroke.

ABCDs of Emergency Cardiac Care

The links in the chain of survival for adults (and children over 12 to 14 years of age) include early access, early cardiopulmonary resuscitation (CPR), early defibrillation, and early advanced cardiac life support.

ABCDs of Emergency Cardiac Care

Risk factors that cannot be modified are called nonmodifiable or fixed risk factors. Examples include:
    Heredity
    Gender
    Race
    Age

ABCDs of Emergency Cardiac Care

List five components of advanced cardiac care.

ABCDs of Emergency Cardiac Care

Describe the electrical phase of cardiopulmonary resuscitation (CPR).

ABCDs of Emergency Cardiac Care

Name the three phases of cardiopulmonary resuscitation (CPR).

ABCDs of Emergency Cardiac Care

What are the first impression ABCs?

ABCDs of Emergency Cardiac Care

Name the four critical tasks of resuscitation.

ABCDs of Emergency Cardiac Care

Name two nonshockable cardiac arrest rhythms.

ABCDs of Emergency Cardiac Care

Name five modifiable risk factors for coronary artery disease.

ABCDs of Emergency Cardiac Care

What is an advance directive?

ABCDs of Emergency Cardiac Care

The electrical phase is the first phase of CPR. It extends from the time of cardiac arrest to about 5 minutes following the arrest. Prompt defibrillation is the most important treatment during this phase.

ABCDs of Emergency Cardiac Care

- Basic life support
- Advanced airway management
- Ventilation support
- Electrocardiogram (ECG)/dysrhythmia recognition
- 12-lead ECG interpretation
- Vascular access and fluid resuscitation
- Electrical therapy including defibrillation, synchronized cardioversion, and pacing
- Giving medications
- Coronary artery bypass, stent insertion, angioplasty

ABCDs of Emergency Cardiac Care

The first impression ABCs are appearance, (work of) breathing, and circulation.

ABCDs of Emergency Cardiac Care

The three phases of CPR are the electrical phase, circulatory (hemodynamic) phase, and metabolic phase. The electrical phase lasts from the time of arrest to about the first 5 minutes after the arrest. The circulatory phase lasts about 5 minutes to 10 or 15 minutes after the arrest. The metabolic phase occurs after about 10 to 15 minutes.

ABCDs of Emergency Cardiac Care

- Asystole
- Pulseless electrical activity

ABCDs of Emergency Cardiac Care

1. Airway management
2. Chest compressions
3. Electrocardiogram (ECG) monitoring and defibrillation
4. Vascular access and drug administration

ABCDs of Emergency Cardiac Care

An advance directive is a written document recording an individual's decision concerning medical treatment that is to be applied (or not applied) in the event of physical or mental inability to communicate these wishes.

ABCDs of Emergency Cardiac Care

- High blood pressure
- Elevated serum cholesterol levels
- Tobacco use
- Diabetes
- Physical inactivity
- Obesity
- Metabolic syndrome

ABCDs of Emergency Cardiac Care

Define cardiac arrest.

ABCDs of Emergency Cardiac Care

Name at least four possible cardiac causes of sudden cardiac death.

ABCDs of Emergency Cardiac Care

What are the components of the primary survey?

ABCDs of Emergency Cardiac Care

Explain each of the following treatment classifications as they are described in the 2005 resuscitation guidelines:
- Class I
- Class IIa
- Class IIb
- Class III
- Indeterminate

ABCDs of Emergency Cardiac Care

Name two shockable cardiac arrest rhythms.

ABCDs of Emergency Cardiac Care

Name at least four possible noncardiac causes of sudden cardiac death.

ABCDs of Emergency Cardiac Care

Explain "contributing risk factors" for coronary artery disease.

ABCDs of Emergency Cardiac Care

During the primary survey, for what length of time should you assess for the presence of a pulse and other signs of circulation?

ABCDs of Emergency Cardiac Care

- Coronary artery disease
- Cardiac dysrhythmias
- Acute myocardial infarction
- Valvular heart disease
- Cardiomyopathy or myocarditis
- Prolonged QT interval
- Congenital heart disease
- Intracardiac tumor
- Wolff-Parkinson-White syndrome
- Pericardial tamponade

ABCDs of Emergency Cardiac Care

Cardiopulmonary (cardiac) arrest is the absence of cardiac mechanical activity, confirmed by the absence of a detectable pulse, unresponsiveness, and apnea or agonal, gasping respiration. The term cardiac arrest is more commonly used than cardiopulmonary arrest when referring to a patient who is not breathing and has no pulse.

ABCDs of Emergency Cardiac Care

The 2005 resuscitation guidelines and treatment recommendations have been classified as follows:
- Class I—Procedure/treatment or diagnostic test/assessment should be performed/administered.
- Class IIa—It is reasonable to perform procedure/administer treatment or perform diagnostic test/assessment.
- Class IIb—Procedure/treatment or diagnostic test/assessment may be considered.
- Class III—Procedure/treatment or diagnostic test/assessment should not be performed/administered. It is not helpful and may be harmful.
- Indeterminate—Research just getting started; continuing area of research; no recommendations until further research (e.g., cannot recommend for or against).

ABCDs of Emergency Cardiac Care

The components of the primary survey are Airway, Breathing, Circulation, and Defibrillation, if necessary (the ABCDs).

ABCDs of Emergency Cardiac Care

- Pulmonary embolism
- Choking and asphyxia
- Drug ingestion (prescribed or nonprescribed)
- Substance abuse
- Stroke
- Hypoxia
- Hypoglycemia
- Alcoholism
- Allergic reactions
- Electrical shock

ABCDs of Emergency Cardiac Care

Pulseless ventricular tachycardia and ventricular fibrillation are "shockable" rhythms. This means that delivering a shock to the heart by means of a defibrillator may result in termination of the rhythm.

ABCDs of Emergency Cardiac Care

A pulse and other signs of circulation should be assessed for up to 10 seconds.

ABCDs of Emergency Cardiac Care

Contributing risk factors are thought to lead to an increased risk of heart disease, but their exact role has not been defined. Examples include stress, inflammatory markers, psychosocial factors (education, family income, employment), and alcohol intake.

Airway Management
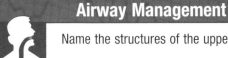

Name the structures of the upper airway.

Airway Management
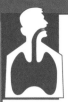

Explain why it is possible to deliver a greater tidal volume using mouth-to-mask ventilation than with bag-mask ventilation.

Airway Management
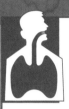

Give three examples of situations in which use of an esophageal detector device (EDD) may yield inaccurate results.

Airway Management
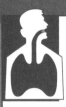

Describe the technique for performing a jaw thrust without head tilt maneuver.

Airway Management

A 47-year-old man has suffered a respiratory arrest. An oral airway is in place. As you begin ventilation with a bag-mask device, you note that there is no rise and fall of the patient's chest with positive-pressure ventilation. What corrective action should be taken at this time?

Airway Management
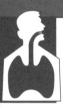

What is the maximum length of time ventilation should be interrupted for an intubation attempt?

Airway Management
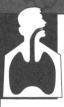

What is a stylet and what is its purpose?

Airway Management

Differentiate between the hard and soft palates of the upper airway.

Airway Management

You can deliver a greater tidal volume to the patient with mouth-to-mask ventilation than with a bag-mask device because both of your hands can be used to secure the mask in place while simultaneously maintaining proper head position. Your vital capacity can also compensate for leaks between the mask and the patient's face, resulting in greater lung ventilation.

Airway Management

The upper airway consists of structures located outside the chest cavity, including the nose and nasal cavities, pharynx, and larynx.

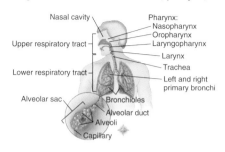

Airway Management

To perform the jaw thrust without head tilt maneuver, place the patient in a supine position. While stabilizing the patient's head in a neutral position, grasp the angles of the patient's lower jaw with both hands, one on each side, and displace the mandible forward.

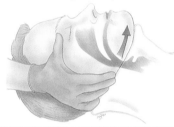

Airway Management

The EDD may be unreliable in patients with chronic obstructive pulmonary disease, morbidly obese patients, or patients in the third trimester of pregnancy—conditions in which negative pressure may cause the trachea to partially collapse and prevent the unrestricted aspiration of air.

The EDD may also be unreliable when there are copious tracheal secretions or in patients with status asthmaticus, because airway secretions or small airway obstruction can prevent air aspiration from the lower airways.

Airway Management

The maximum length of time ventilation should be interrupted for an intubation attempt is 30 seconds.

Airway Management

If the chest does not rise and fall with bag-mask ventilation, reassess.
- Reassess head position; reposition the airway, and try again to ventilate.
- Inadequate tidal volume delivery may be the result of an improper mask seal or incomplete bag compression.
- If air is escaping from under the mask, reposition your fingers and the mask.
- Reevaluate the effectiveness of bag compression.
- Check for an airway obstruction:
  - Lift the jaw.
  - Suction the airway as needed.

If the chest still does not rise, select an alternative method of positive-pressure ventilation (such as a pocket mask or an automatic transport ventilator).

Airway Management

The hard palate is the bony portion of the roof of the mouth that forms the floor of the nasal cavity. The soft palate is the back part of the roof of the mouth that is made up of mucous membrane, muscular fibers, and mucous glands.

Airway Management

A stylet is a plastic-coated wire that may be inserted into an endotracheal tube before an endotracheal intubation attempt. It is used to mold and maintain the shape of the tube. The tip of the stylet must be recessed at least 1/2 inch from the end of the endotracheal tube to avoid trauma to the airway structures.

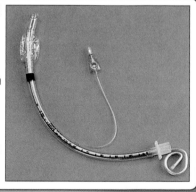

Airway Management

Describe an Esophageal-Tracheal Combitube (ETC).

Airway Management

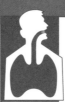

Name four signs of respiratory distress.

Airway Management

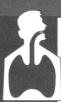

Explain how you would locate the correct position for application of cricoid pressure.

Airway Management

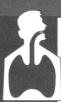

Describe the advantages of the airway adjunct shown here.

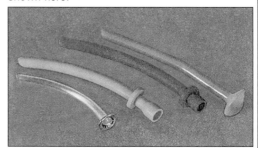

Airway Management

Name two advantages of pulse oximetry.

Airway Management

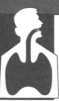

What is the purpose of cricoid pressure (the Sellick maneuver)? How is this technique performed?

Airway Management

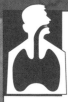

Describe two methods for insertion of an oral airway in an adult.

Airway Management

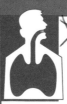

What is the average endotracheal tube size for
- An adult woman?
- An adult man?

Airway Management

There are many signs of respiratory distress, including the following:
- Nasal flaring
- Tracheal tugging
- Jugular venous distention
- Inability to speak in full sentences
- Confusion, agitation, combativeness
- Dyspnea (difficult or labored breathing)
- Retractions
- Use of accessory muscles of respiration

Airway Management

The Combitube is a dual-lumen tube with two balloon cuffs. The proximal (pharyngeal) balloon is located near the halfway point of the tube and is considerably larger than the distal cuff. When inflated, the balloon fills the space between the base of the tongue and the soft palate, anchoring the Combitube into position, and isolating the oropharynx from the hypopharynx.

When both balloon cuffs are inflated, an airtight pocket is created in the pharynx between the upper portion of the esophagus (blocked by a balloon) and the area behind the tongue and molars (blocked by the other balloon). Air can escape only into the trachea and then to the lungs.

Airway Management

Nasal airway advantages include the following:
- Provides patent airway
- Tolerated by responsive patients
- Does not require the patient's mouth to be open

Airway Management

To better understand the anatomy, try this on yourself.

Locate your thyroid cartilage (Adam's apple). It is the largest and most superior cartilage in the neck and is shaped like a shield. As you slide your fingers slowly down this cartilage, you will reach a soft membranous structure. This is the cricothyroid membrane. Just below the cricothyroid membrane is another firm structure. This is the cricoid cartilage, where cricoid pressure is applied.

The thyroid cartilage is more pronounced in adult men than in adult women. In women, it may be easier to locate the sternal notch and move your fingers slowly toward the head. The first hard structure you palpate is the cricoid cartilage.

Airway Management

Cricoid pressure (the Sellick maneuver) may be applied to minimize gastric distention and aspiration. Locate the cricoid cartilage and apply firm pressure on the cricoid cartilage with your thumb and index or middle finger, just lateral to midline.

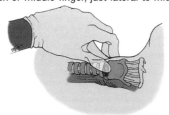

Airway Management

- Painless
- Noninvasive
- Does not require drawing or handling of blood
- Can provide a continuous measurement of oxygenation

Airway Management

Endotracheal (ET) tubes are measured in millimeters by their internal diameter (ID) and external diameter (OD).

Average ET tube sizes are as follows:
- Adult woman: 7.0 to 8.0 mm ID
- Adult man: 8.0 to 8.5 mm ID

Airway Management

The oral airway is inserted upside down (with the tip pointing toward the roof of the mouth). When the distal end reaches the posterior wall of the pharynx, the airway is rotated 180 degrees and slipped behind the tongue into the posterior pharynx.

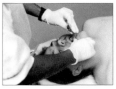

A tongue blade may be used to depress the tongue. If this method is used, the oral airway is inserted right side up into the oropharynx.

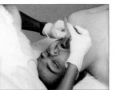

Airway Management

What percentage of oxygen can be delivered by means of a nasal cannula (prongs) connected to oxygen at 1 to 6 L/min?

Airway Management

Name four advantages of mouth-to-mask ventilation.

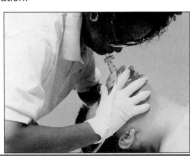

Airway Management

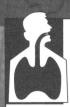

Name three possible complications of cricoid pressure.

Airway Management

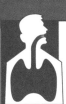

A 78-year-old woman experienced a respiratory arrest and was subsequently intubated. You note that there is an absence of chest wall movement with positive-pressure ventilation and you are unable to auscultate breath sounds on either side of the chest. What is the most likely cause of this situation? What corrective action will you initiate?

Airway Management

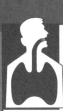

What is the minimum oxygen flow rate that should be used with a simple face mask?

Airway Management

Name four advantages of using a nasal cannula for oxygen delivery.

Airway Management

Name five possible complications of endotracheal intubation.

Airway Management

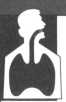

A 64-year-old man in respiratory failure has just been intubated. How will you confirm correct placement of the endotracheal (ET) tube?

Airway Management

- Aesthetically more acceptable than mouth-to-mouth ventilation
- Easy to teach and learn
- Physical barrier between rescuer and patient's nose, mouth, and secretions
- If patient resumes spontaneous breathing, can be used as a simple face mask
- Greater tidal volume can be delivered with mouth-to-mask ventilation than with a bag-mask device
- Rescuer can feel compliance of patient's lungs

Airway Management

A nasal cannula can deliver an oxygen concentration of 25% to 45% at a flow rate of 1 to 6 L/min. The formula to calculate the O_2 percentage at a given liter flow is 21% (room air) + 4 × oxygen flow in L/min.

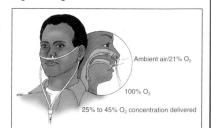

- 1 L/min = 25%
- 2 L/min = 29%
- 3 L/min = 33%
- 4 L/min = 37%
- 5 L/min = 41%
- 6 L/min = 45%

Airway Management

The endotracheal tube is most likely in the esophagus. Deflate the endotracheal tube cuff and remove the endotracheal tube. Oxygenate the patient before attempting another intubation.

Airway Management

- Laryngeal trauma with excessive force
- Esophageal rupture from unrelieved high gastric pressures
- If active regurgitation occurs while performing cricoid pressure, release pressure to avoid rupture of the stomach or esophagus
- In small children, use of excessive pressure may obstruct the trachea

Airway Management

- Comfortable, well tolerated by most patients
- Does not interfere with patient assessment or impede patient communication with health care personnel
- Allows for talking and eating
- No rebreathing of expired air
- Can be used with mouth breathers
- Useful in patients predisposed to carbon dioxide retention
- Can be used for patients who require oxygen but cannot tolerate a nonrebreather mask

Airway Management

When using a simple face mask, the oxygen flow rate must be greater than 5 to 6 L/min to flush the accumulation of the patient's exhaled carbon dioxide from the mask.

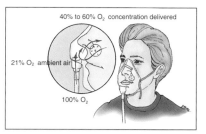

Airway Management

Primary methods
- Visualizing passage of ET tube between the vocal cords
- Auscultating presence of bilateral breath sounds
- Confirming absence of sounds over epigastrium during ventilation
- Adequate chest rise with each ventilation
- Absence of vocal sounds after placement of ET tube

Secondary methods
- Monitoring for changes in the color (colorimetric device) or number (digital device) on an end-tidal CO_2 detector
- Verification by an esophageal detector device
- Chest x-ray

Airway Management

- Bleeding
- Laryngospasm
- Vocal cord damage
- Mucosal necrosis
- Barotrauma
- Aspiration
- Cuff leak
- Esophageal intubation
- Right mainstem intubation

Airway Management

Name three advantages of automatic transport ventilators.

Airway Management

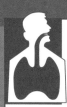

Name three situations in which exhaled carbon dioxide monitoring is commonly performed.

Airway Management

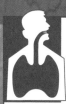

When used during a resuscitation effort, a bag-mask device should not possess a pop-off (pressure-release) valve. What is the reason for this?

Airway Management

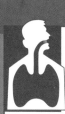

Name four advantages of the Esophageal-Tracheal Combitube.

Airway Management

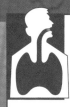

Name two indications for use of the airway adjunct shown here.

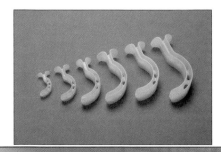

Airway Management

What is the maximum length of time an adult patient should be suctioned at one time?

Airway Management

An endotracheal intubation attempt should not take more than 30 seconds. At what point does this 30-second interval begin and end?

Airway Management

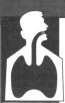

A 65-year-old man is found unresponsive in bed. Trauma is not suspected. How should you open this patient's airway?

Airway Management

Exhaled CO_2 monitoring is commonly used in the following situations:
- Assessment of conscious sedation safety
- Evaluation of mechanical ventilation and resuscitation efforts
- Verification of endotracheal (ET) tube placement
- Continuous monitoring of ET tube position
- Monitoring of exhaled CO_2 levels in patients with suspected increased intracranial pressure

Airway Management

- Frees the rescuer for other tasks when used in intubated patients.
- In patients who are not intubated, the rescuer has both hands free for mask application and airway maintenance.
- Cricoid pressure can be applied with one hand while the other seals the mask on the face.
- Once set, provides a specific tidal volume, respiratory rate, and minute volume.

Airway Management

- Minimal training and retraining required
- Visualization of the upper airway or use of special equipment not required for insertion
- Reasonable technique for use in suspected neck injury since the head does not need to be hyperextended
- Because of the oropharyngeal balloon, the need for a face mask is eliminated
- Can provide an open airway with either esophageal or tracheal placement
- If placed in the esophagus, allows suctioning of gastric contents without interruption of ventilation
- Reduces risk of aspiration of gastric contents

Airway Management

Ventilation of patients in cardiac arrest often requires higher than usual airway pressures. Higher than usual ventilation pressures may also be needed in situations involving near-drowning, pulmonary edema, and asthma. To effectively ventilate a patient in these situations, the pressures needed for ventilation may exceed the limits of the pop-off valve. Thus a pop-off valve may prevent generation of sufficient tidal volume to overcome the increase in airway resistance. Disabling the pop-off valve, or using a bag-mask device with no pop-off valve, helps ensure delivery of adequate tidal volumes to the patient during resuscitation. To disable a pop-off valve, depress the valve with a finger during ventilation or twist the pop-off valve into the closed position.

Airway Management

Limit suctioning to no more than 10 to 15 seconds. Be sure to oxygenate the patient before and after suctioning.

Airway Management

Indications for use of an oral airway include the following:
- To aid in maintaining an open airway in an unresponsive patient who is not intubated
- To aid in maintaining an open airway in an unresponsive patient with no gag reflex that is being ventilated with a bag-mask or other positive-pressure device
- May be used as a bite block after insertion of an endotracheal tube or oral gastric tube
Note: An oral airway does not provide protection against aspiration.

Airway Management

The patient's airway should be opened using a head-tilt/chin-lift. Place one of your hands on the patient's forehead and apply firm downward pressure with your palm to tilt the patient's head back. Place the tips of the fingers of your other hand under the bony part of the patient's chin and gently lift the jaw forward.

Airway Management

The 30-second interval begins when ventilation of the patient ceases to allow insertion of the laryngoscope blade into the patient's mouth and ends when the patient is reventilated on placement of the endotracheal tube.

Airway Management

Name three possible complications of suctioning.

Airway Management

Name two disadvantages of the nasal airway.

Airway Management

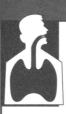

Name two advantages of ventilation with the bag-mask device.

Airway Management

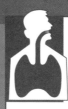

When using a pocket mask, an oxygen flow rate of 10 L/min will provide approximately what percentage of an inspired oxygen concentration?

Airway Management

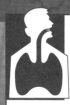

You are preparing to insert a nasal airway. How will you determine the proper airway size for your patient?

Airway Management

Name two types of suction catheters.

Airway Management

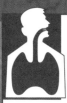

A 61-year-old man has experienced a respiratory arrest. An endotracheal tube has been correctly placed, and you are preparing to ventilate the patient with a bag-mask device. What oxygen liter flow should be used when ventilating the patient with the device?

Airway Management

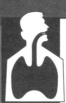

You are intubating a patient in cardiac arrest and have visualized the vocal cords. How far should the endotracheal tube be advanced beyond the vocal cords?

Airway Management

Disadvantages of the nasal airway include the following:
- Improper technique may result in severe bleeding
- Resulting epistaxis may be difficult to control
- Does not protect the lower airway from aspiration
- May be difficult to insert if nasal damage (new or old) is present

Airway Management

- Hypoxia
- Dysrhythmias
- Increased intracranial pressure
- Local swelling
- Hemorrhage
- Tracheal ulceration
- Tracheal infection
- Bronchospasm
- Bradycardia and hypotension caused by vagal stimulation

Airway Management

When using a pocket mask, an oxygen flow rate of 10 L/min will provide an inspired oxygen concentration of about 50%.

Airway Management

- Provides a means for delivery of an oxygen-enriched mixture to the patient
- Conveys a sense of compliance of patient's lungs to the bag-mask operator
- Provides a means for immediate ventilatory support
- Can be used with the spontaneously breathing patient and the apneic patient

Airway Management

- Soft catheters; also called "whistle-tip" or "French" catheters
- Rigid catheters; also called "hard," "tonsil tip," or "Yankauer" catheters

Airway Management

Proper airway size is determined by holding the device against the side of the patient's face and selecting an airway that extends from the tip of the nose to the angle of the jaw or the tip of the ear.

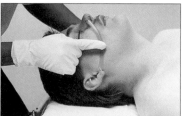

Airway Management

The proximal end of the endotracheal tube cuff should be advanced about 1 to 2.5 cm (1/2 to 1 inch) beyond the vocal cords.

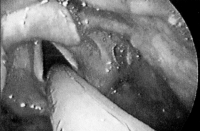

Airway Management

The patient should be ventilated with the bag-mask device (with a reservoir) connected to supplemental oxygen with at least 10 to 15 L/min flow.

Airway Management

Name two advantages associated with the use of an oral airway.

Airway Management

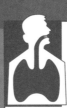

Name three indications for use of the Esophageal-Tracheal Combitube (ETC).

Airway Management

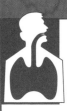

The "BURP" technique may be useful during endotracheal intubation. Describe this technique.

Airway Management

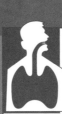

What is the purpose of a laryngoscope?

Airway Management

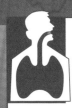

Name two indications for use of a nasal airway.

Airway Management

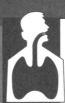

You are preparing to suction a patient with an orotracheal tube in place. What type of suction catheter should be used? How far should the catheter be inserted?

Airway Management

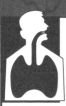

A 78-year-old woman has experienced a respiratory arrest. You have intubated the patient and note that lung sounds are now present on the right but diminished on the left. What is the most likely cause of this situation? What corrective action will you initiate?

Airway Management

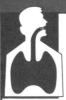

You are preparing to ventilate a patient with a bag-mask device. How will you determine appropriate face mask size for the patient?

Airway Management

- Difficult face mask fit (beards, absence of teeth)
- Patient in whom intubation has been unsuccessful and ventilation is difficult
- Patient in whom airway management is necessary but health care provider is untrained in technique of visualized orotracheal intubation
- Whenever a direct view of the vocal cords is difficult or impossible (view obscured by edema, blood, tissue damage, or anatomic distortion)

Airway Management

An oral airway
- Holds the tongue away from the posterior wall of the pharynx
- Is easily placed
- Permits suctioning on either side of the device
- May serve as an effective bite block in intubated patients, preventing biting of the endotracheal tube

Airway Management

A laryngoscope consists of a handle and blade used for examining the interior of the larynx. The handle contains batteries for the light source. The laryngoscope handle attaches to a blade with a bulb at the distal tip. The laryngoscope:
- Permits direct visualization of the vocal cords/glottis
- Is used to align the structures of the upper airway to facilitate endotracheal intubation

Airway Management

The "BURP" (Backward, Upward, Rightward Pressure) technique may be used to facilitate visualization of the vocal cords. With this maneuver, the larynx is displaced in three specific directions: (1) posteriorly against the cervical vertebrae, (2) superiorly as possible, and (3) slightly laterally to the right. This maneuver has been shown to improve visualization of the larynx more easily than simple back pressure on the larynx (cricoid pressure) because the back-up-right pressure moves the larynx back to the position from which it was displaced by a right-handed (held in operator's left hand) laryngoscope.

Airway Management

A soft suction catheter can be inserted into the nares, oropharynx, or nasopharynx; through an oral or nasal airway; or through an endotracheal tube. To measure the correct length to insert the suction catheter for orotracheal suctioning, measure the distance from the mouth to the ear and add the distance from the ear to the sternal notch.

Airway Management

A nasal airway may be used to aid in maintaining an open airway when use of an oral airway is contraindicated or impossible:
- Trismus (spasm of the muscles used to grind, crush, and chew food)
- Biting
- Clenched jaws or teeth

Airway Management

Selection of a mask of proper size is essential to ensuring a good seal. A mask of correct size should extend from the bridge of the nose to the groove between the lower lip and chin.

If the mask is not properly positioned and a tight seal maintained, air will leak from between the mask and the patient's face, resulting in less tidal volume delivery to the patient.

Airway Management

The endotracheal tube is most likely in the right mainstem bronchus. Deflate the endotracheal tube cuff and pull back the tube slightly. Reinflate the endotracheal tube cuff and reassess lung sounds.

Airway Management

State the equipment needed for endotracheal intubation.

Airway Management

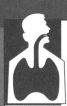

You have intubated a patient in cardiopulmonary arrest. Name two possible consequences of unrecognized esophageal intubation.

Airway Management

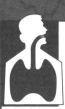

Locate the following on this illustration:
- Epiglottis
- Base of the tongue
- Glottic opening

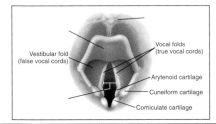

Vestibular fold
(false vocal cords)

Vocal folds
(true vocal cords)

Arytenoid cartilage

Cuneiform cartilage

Corniculate cartilage

Airway Management

How is proper placement of a laryngeal mask airway (LMA) confirmed?

Airway Management

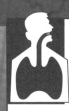

Name two indications for endotracheal intubation.

Airway Management

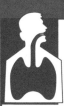

Name three advantages for using a laryngeal mask airway.

Airway Management

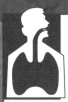

Name two disadvantages of bag-mask ventilation.

Airway Management

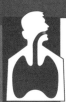

What is the "sniffing" position?

Airway Management

- Cerebral hypoxia
- Brain damage
- Death

Airway Management

- Laryngoscope handle
- Laryngoscope blades
- Extra batteries
- Endotracheal (ET) tubes of various sizes
- 10 mL syringe for inflation of the ET tube cuff (if present)
- Stylet
- Bag-mask device (mask removed after intubation) with supplemental oxygen and reservoir
- Suction equipment
- Commercial tube-holder or tape
- Water-soluble lubricant
- Bite-block or oral airway
- Exhaled CO_2 detector and/or esophageal detector device

Airway Management

Confirm proper placement of an LMA by
- Auscultation
- Observing chest rise
- Use of an exhaled CO_2 detector

  Esophageal detector devices should not be used with LMAs, because a properly positioned LMA lies in the upper portion of the esophagus.

Airway Management

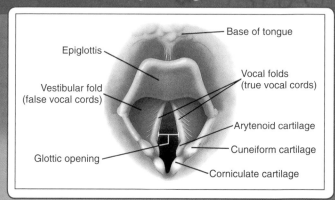

Airway Management

- Can be quickly inserted to provide ventilation when bag-mask ventilation is not sufficient and endotracheal intubation cannot be readily accomplished
- Tidal volume delivered may be greater when using the LMA than with face mask ventilation
- Less gastric insufflation than with bag-mask ventilation
- Provides ventilation equivalent to the tracheal tube
- Training simpler than with tracheal intubation
- Unaffected by anatomic factors (e.g., beard, absence of teeth)
- No risk of esophageal or bronchial intubation
- When compared to tracheal intubation, less potential for trauma from direct laryngoscopy and tracheal intubation
- Less coughing, laryngeal spasm, sore throat, and voice changes than with tracheal intubation

Airway Management

Indications for endotracheal intubation include the following:
- Cardiac arrest with ongoing chest compressions
- Inability of the conscious patient to ventilate adequately
- Inability of the patient to protect his or her own airway (coma, areflexia, cardiac arrest)
- Inability of the rescuer to ventilate the unconscious patient with conventional methods.

Airway Management

In the "sniffing" position, the neck is flexed at the fifth and sixth cervical vertebrae, and the head is extended at the first and second cervical vertebrae. This position aligns the axes of the mouth, pharynx, and trachea for endotracheal intubation. The sniffing position is not used in cases of suspected trauma.

Airway Management

- Inability to provide adequate ventilatory volumes
- Should only be used by trained operators
- Difficult to use by inexperienced operators
- Gastric distention

Rhythm Recognition

Label the following coronary arteries:
- Circumflex
- Posterior descending
- Anterior descending
- Marginal
- Right coronary artery
- Left main coronary artery

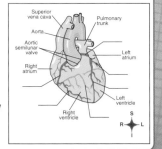

Rhythm Recognition

Locate the following parts of the conduction system on this illustration:
- Right bundle branch
- Left bundle branch
- AV node
- SA node
- Purkinje fibers
- Bundle of His

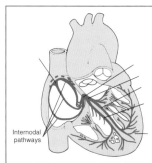

Rhythm Recognition

What complications may result from occlusion of the right coronary artery?

Rhythm Recognition

Label each of the left and right chest leads on this illustration.

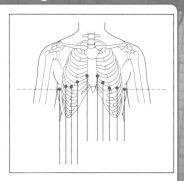

Rhythm Recognition

Depolarization and repolarization are changes that occur in the heart when an impulse forms and spreads throughout the myocardium. These changes occur due to the movement of ions across the cell membrane. Do these illustrations reflect depolarization or repolarization?

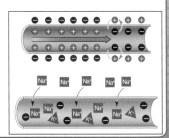

Rhythm Recognition

Name the lead illustrated here.

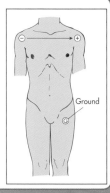

Rhythm Recognition

Explain the significance of each of the numbers illustrated and their relationship to ventricular depolarization or repolarization.

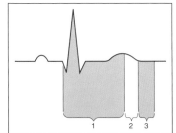

Rhythm Recognition

Label the following on this illustration:
- Voltage (amplitude) axis
- Time axis
- P wave, Q wave, R wave, S wave, T wave
- PR interval and its normal duration
- QRS duration and its normal value
- S-T segment
- Q-T interval and its normal duration

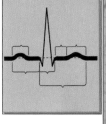

Rhythm Recognition

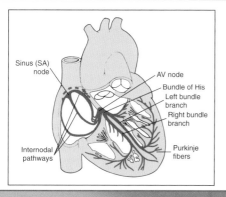

Sinus (SA) node
AV node
Bundle of His
Left bundle branch
Right bundle branch
Internodal pathways
Purkinje fibers

Rhythm Recognition

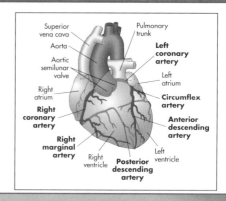

Superior vena cava
Aorta
Aortic semilunar valve
Right atrium
Right coronary artery
Right marginal artery
Right ventricle
Posterior descending artery
Pulmonary trunk
Left coronary artery
Left atrium
Circumflex artery
Anterior descending artery
Left ventricle

Rhythm Recognition

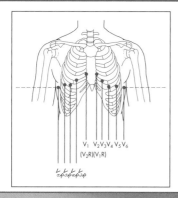

V₁ V₂V₃V₄ V₅V₆
(V₂R)(V₁R)

Rhythm Recognition

The right coronary artery (RCA) supplies the inferior wall of the left ventricle. The marginal branch supplies the right atrium and right ventricle. In 50% to 60% of individuals, a branch of the RCA supplies the sinoatrial node. In 85% to 90% of hearts, the RCA also branches into the atrioventricular (AV) node artery. Occlusion of the RCA can result in inferior wall myocardial infarction (MI) (and, in some patients, posterior MI), and disturbances in AV nodal conduction.

Rhythm Recognition

The electrode placement shown is consistent with lead I. Lead I records the difference in electrical potential between the left arm (+) and right arm (−) electrodes. The positive electrode is placed just below the left clavicle (or on the left arm) and the negative electrode is placed just below the right clavicle (or on the right arm). The third electrode is a ground that minimizes electrical activity from other sources.

Rhythm Recognition

These illustrations reflect depolarization. When the cardiac muscle cell is stimulated, the cell is said to depolarize. The inside of the cell becomes more positive because of the entry of sodium (Na⁺) ions into the cell through Na⁺ membrane channels. Thus depolarization occurs because of the inward diffusion of Na⁺.

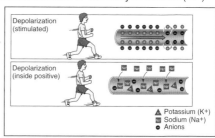

Depolarization (stimulated)
Depolarization (inside positive)
▲ Potassium (K+)
Sodium (Na+)
● Anions

Rhythm Recognition

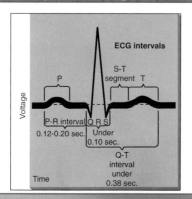

ECG intervals
Voltage
P
S-T segment
T
P-R interval
0.12-0.20 sec.
Q R S
Under 0.10 sec.
Q-T interval under 0.38 sec.
Time

Rhythm Recognition

1 = Absolute refractory period
   Onset of QRS complex to approximately peak of T wave
   Cardiac cells cannot be stimulated to conduct an electrical impulse, no matter how strong the stimulus
2 = Relative refractory period
   Corresponds with the downslope of the T wave
   Cardiac cells can be stimulated to depolarize if the stimulus is strong enough
3 = Supernormal period
   Corresponds with the end of the T wave
   A weaker than normal stimulus can cause depolarization of cardiac cells

Rhythm Recognition

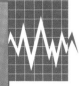

One method used to calculate heart rate requires determining the number of large boxes between two consecutive R waves (ventricular rate) or P waves (atrial rate). Complete the following table.

# of large boxes	Heart rate (beats/min)	# of large boxes	Heart rate (beats/min)
1		6	
2		7	
3		8	
4		9	
5		10	

Rhythm Recognition

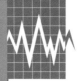

What area(s) of the heart is/are supplied by the left circumflex coronary artery?

Rhythm Recognition

Complete the following table regarding standard limb leads.

Lead	Positive electrode position	Negative electrode position	Heart surface viewed
I			
II			
III			

Rhythm Recognition

Name four types of vagal maneuvers.

Rhythm Recognition

Name the lead illustrated here.

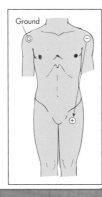

Ground

Rhythm Recognition

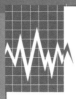

What is the significance of the absolute refractory period?

Rhythm Recognition

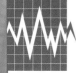

Define each of the following terms as they relate to the ECG:
- Waveform
- Segment
- Interval
- Complex

Rhythm Recognition

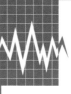

Describe the primary function of the atrioventricular (AV) node.

Rhythm Recognition

The left circumflex coronary artery supplies the lateral wall of the left ventricle. Occlusion can result in a lateral wall myocardial infarction (MI).

In some patients, the circumflex artery may also supply the inferior portion of the left ventricle. A posterior wall MI may occur because of occlusion of the right coronary artery or the left circumflex artery.

Rhythm Recognition

# of large boxes	Heart rate (beats/min)	# of large boxes	Heart rate (beats/min)
1	300	6	50
2	150	7	43
3	100	8	38
4	75	9	33
5	60	10	30

Rhythm Recognition

Examples of vagal maneuvers:
- Valsalva's maneuver (bearing down, breath holding)
- Coughing
- Squatting
- Gagging
- Carotid sinus pressure
- Application of a cold stimulus to the patient's face

Rhythm Recognition

Lead	Positive electrode position	Negative electrode position	Heart surface viewed
I	Left arm	Right arm	Lateral
II	Left leg	Right arm	Inferior
III	Left leg	Left arm	Inferior

Rhythm Recognition

The absolute refractory period (also known as the effective refractory period) extends from the onset of the QRS complex to approximately the peak of the T wave. During this period, cardiac cells have not yet repolarized and, no matter how strong a stimulus, cannot be stimulated to depolarize.

Rhythm Recognition

The electrode placement shown is consistent with lead III.

Rhythm Recognition

The main function of the AV node is to delay the electrical impulse it receives from the SA node. This allows the atria to contract and empty blood into the ventricles, promoting adequate ventricular filling before the next contraction of the ventricles.

Rhythm Recognition

- Waveform: Movement away from the baseline in either a positive or negative direction
- Segment: A line between waveforms; named by the waveform that precedes or follows it
- Interval: A waveform and a segment
- Complex: Several waveforms

Rhythm Recognition

What is the cardiac action potential?

Rhythm Recognition

Describe how carotid sinus pressure is performed.

Rhythm Recognition

Describe normal electrical flow through the heart.

Rhythm Recognition

Is depolarization the same as contraction?

Rhythm Recognition

What is the first positive deflection seen after the P wave on the ECG, and what does it represent?

Rhythm Recognition

How would you determine if the atrial rhythm on a rhythm strip was regular or irregular?

Rhythm Recognition

Name the lead illustrated here.

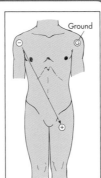

Ground

Rhythm Recognition

What is the normal pacemaker of the heart and where is it located?

Rhythm Recognition

- Carotid sinus pressure should be avoided in older patients and in patients with carotid artery bruits. Auscultate to ensure carotid bruits are absent.
- Establish venous access and ensure emergency medications are immediately available. Carotid sinus pressure should be performed while continuously monitoring the ECG.
- Turn the patient's head to the left and apply firm pressure on the right carotid bifurcation near the angle of the jaw for 5 seconds or less. If unsuccessful, the procedure may be repeated with a "massaging" motion lasting 5 seconds or less. Simultaneous, bilateral carotid pressure should *never* be performed.

Rhythm Recognition

Electrical impulses occur as the result of brief but rapid flow of positively charged ions back and forth across the cell membrane. The cardiac action potential is an illustration of the changes in the membrane potential of a cardiac cell during depolarization and repolarization.

Rhythm Recognition

No. Depolarization is an electrical event, whereas contraction is a mechanical event. We expect depolarization to result in stimulation of the myocardial working cells (mechanical cells) to contract, thus producing a pulse; however, it is possible for electrical activity to occur without a mechanical response (pulse). When organized electrical activity with an adequate rate is viewed on the cardiac monitor and a pulse cannot be obtained, we term the clinical situation Pulseless Electrical Activity (PEA).

Rhythm Recognition

The impulse originates in the SA node and travels to the AV node, to the bundle of His, to the left and right bundle branches, and then to the Purkinje fibers where the mechanical cells are stimulated.

Rhythm Recognition

To determine if the atrial rhythm is regular or irregular, measure the distance between two consecutive P-P intervals and compare that distance with another P-P interval. If the atrial rhythm is regular, the P-P intervals will measure the same.

Rhythm Recognition

The first positive deflection seen after the P wave on the ECG is the R wave. The QRS complex represents ventricular depolarization.

Rhythm Recognition

The normal pacemaker of the heart is the sinoatrial (SA) node because it depolarizes more rapidly than any other part of the cardiac conduction system.

The SA node is located at the junction of the superior vena cava and right atrium.

Rhythm Recognition

The electrode placement shown is consistent with lead II. Lead II records the difference in electrical potential between the left leg (+) and right arm (−) electrodes. The positive electrode is placed below the left pectoral muscle (or on the left leg) and the negative electrode is placed just below the right clavicle (or on the right arm). The third electrode is a ground that minimizes electrical activity from other sources.

Rhythm Recognition

Name and describe the four properties of cardiac cells.

Rhythm Recognition

How does complete (third-degree) AV block differ from second-degree AV block, type I?

Rhythm Recognition

Describe the PR intervals in second-degree AV block, type I and second-degree AV block, type II.

Rhythm Recognition

How would you determine if the ventricular rhythm on a rhythm strip was regular or irregular?

Rhythm Recognition

Even properly performed carotid sinus pressure may result in complications. Name two possible complications of this procedure.

Rhythm Recognition

What does the QT interval represent and how is it measured?

Rhythm Recognition

Name at least four possible causes of sinus tachycardia.

Rhythm Recognition

Explain how baseline wander can affect ST-segment analysis.

Rhythm Recognition

In complete (third-degree) AV block:
- There is a regular atrial and ventricular rhythm.
- There is no PR interval because the atria and ventricles beat independently of each other.

In second-degree AV block, type I (Wenckebach):
- The atrial rhythm is regular.
- The ventricular rhythm is irregular.
- The PR interval lengthens until a P wave appears with no QRS.

Rhythm Recognition

Automaticity: Ability of cardiac pacemaker cells to spontaneously initiate an electrical impulse without being stimulated from another source (such as a nerve)

Excitability: Ability of cardiac muscle cells to respond to an outside stimulus

Conductivity: Ability of a cardiac cell to receive an electrical stimulus and conduct that impulse to an adjacent cardiac cell

Contractility: Ability of cardiac cells to shorten, causing cardiac muscle contraction in response to an electrical stimulus

Rhythm Recognition

To determine if the ventricular rhythm is regular or irregular, measure the distance between two consecutive R-R intervals and compare that distance with another R-R interval. If the ventricular rhythm is regular, the R-R intervals will measure the same.

Rhythm Recognition

In second-degree AV block, type I (Wenckebach, Mobitz I), the PR intervals lengthen until a P wave appears without a QRS.

In second-degree AV block, type II (Mobitz II), the PR interval may be normal or prolonged, but will measure the same for each conducted QRS.

Rhythm Recognition

- The QT interval represents total ventricular activity (the time required for ventricular depolarization and repolarization to take place).
- The QT interval is measured from the beginning of the QRS complex to the end of the T wave.

Rhythm Recognition

Possible complications of carotid sinus pressure include the following:
- Bradycardia
- AV blocks
- Asystole
- Ventricular dysrhythmias
- Syncope, seizures, or CVA as a result of interference with the cerebral circulation

Rhythm Recognition

When the position of the baseline is in a state of flux, ST-segment analysis is very difficult. As the baseline wanders, the isoelectric point changes from moment to moment. In this situation, the J point, though it may have been isoelectric when inscribed, can appear elevated above the PR and TP segments when in fact they are not. Therefore, be very cautious about analyzing ST-segment elevation in leads with a wandering baseline. If an ECG is being obtained via a standard monitor, wait until the tracing is centered for several beats before moving to the next lead.

Rhythm Recognition

- Fever
- Anxiety
- Congestive heart failure
- Infection
- Shock
- Dehydration
- Fright
- Administration of medications such as epinephrine, atropine, dopamine, and dobutamine
- Caffeine-containing beverages, nicotine, and cocaine
- Pain
- Hypoxia
- Acute myocardial infarction
- Sympathetic stimulation
- Hypovolemia
- Exercise

Rhythm Recognition

What is the atrioventricular (AV) junction?

Rhythm Recognition

What is the significance of the relative refractory period?

Rhythm Recognition

What does the PR interval represent and how is it measured?

Rhythm Recognition

What portion of the ECG represents ventricular repolarization?

Rhythm Recognition

Name the valve that separates the right ventricle from the right atrium.

Rhythm Recognition

What is the normal duration of the PR interval?

Rhythm Recognition

What is artifact on an ECG tracing?

Rhythm Recognition

Describe the PR interval in a junctional rhythm.

The relative refractory period (also known as the vulnerable period) corresponds with the downslope of the T wave. During this period most, but not all, cardiac cells have repolarized and can be stimulated to depolarize if a stimulus is strong enough.

The AV junction is the AV node and the nonbranching portion of the bundle of His. The AV node does not contain pacemaker cells. The pacemaker cells in the AV junction are located near the nonbranching portion of the bundle of His.

The T wave represents ventricular repolarization.

The P wave + the PR segment = the PR interval. The PR interval reflects depolarization of the right and left atria (P wave) and the spread of the impulse through the AV node, bundle of His, bundle branches, and Purkinje fibers (PR segment). The PR interval is measured from the beginning of the P wave to the beginning of the QRS complex.

The PR interval normally measures 0.12 to 0.20 second.

The tricuspid valve separates the right atrium and right ventricle.

- If a P wave precedes the QRS complex, the PR interval will typically be less than 0.12 second.
- If a P wave occurs during the QRS complex or after it, there will be no PR interval.

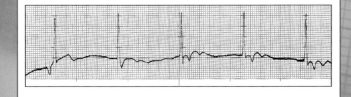

Artifact is distortion of an ECG tracing by electrical activity that is noncardiac in origin.

Rhythm Recognition

State the characteristics of third-degree (complete) AV block.

Rhythm Recognition

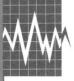

State the ECG characteristics of atrial flutter.

Rhythm Recognition

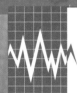

This rhythm strip is from 35-year-old woman complaining of chest pain and palpitations. Identify the rhythm (lead II).

Rhythm Recognition

This rhythm strip is from an 86-year-old woman who experienced a cardiopulmonary arrest. The initial rhythm was asystole. The following rhythm resulted after IV administration of epinephrine and atropine. Identify the rhythm (lead III).

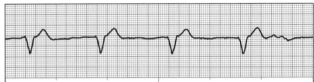

Rhythm Recognition

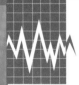

Where is the level of AV block in:
- Second-degree AV block, type I?
- Second-degree AV block, type II?
- Complete (third-degree) AV block?

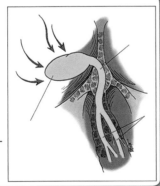

Rhythm Recognition

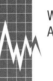

What are the ECG characteristics of first-degree AV block?

Rhythm Recognition

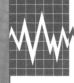

A rhythm that is ventricular in origin has an intrinsic rate of __ beats/min and is called a(n) __.

If the ventricular rate increases to a rate of 40 to 100 beats/min the rhythm is called a(n)

__

If the ventricular rate exceeds 100 beats/min it is called __.

Rhythm Recognition

These rhythm strips are from a 63-year-old man complaining of epigastric pain. Identify the rhythm.

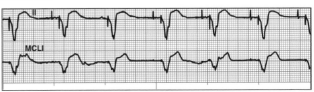

MCLI

Rhythm Recognition

Characteristics of atrial flutter:
- Rate: Atrial rate 250 to 450/minute; ventricular rate variable—determined by AV blockade; the ventricular rate will usually not exceed 180 beats/minute because of the intrinsic conduction rate of the AV junction
- Rhythm: Atrial regular, ventricular regular or irregular depending on AV conduction/blockade
- P waves: No identifiable P waves; saw-toothed "flutter" waves are present
- PR interval: Not measurable
- QRS: Usually 0.10 second in duration or less but may be widened if flutter waves are buried in the QRS complex or an intraventricular conduction delay exists

Rhythm Recognition

Third-degree (complete) AV block:
- More P waves than QRS complexes
- P waves occur regularly
- Regular ventricular rhythm
- No PR interval because the atria and ventricles beat independently of each other
- QRS may be wide or narrow depending on the location of the escape pacemaker and the condition of the ventricular conduction system.

Rhythm Recognition

Idioventricular rhythm (IVR) (also called ventricular escape rhythm)
- Ventricular rhythm: Regular
- Ventricular rate: 40/min
- Atrial rhythm: None
- Atrial rate: None
- PRI: None
- QRS: 0.18 second

Rhythm Recognition

Narrow-QRS tachycardia (SVT) with ST-segment depression
- Ventricular rhythm: Regular
- Ventricular rate: 188/min
- Atrial rhythm: Unable to determine
- Atrial rate: Unable to determine
- PRI: Unable to determine
- QRS: 0.06 second

Rhythm Recognition

Characteristics of first-degree AV block:
- Rate: Atrial and ventricular within normal limits and the same
- Rhythm: Atrial and ventricular regular
- P waves: Normal in size and configuration; one P wave before each QRS
- PR interval: Prolonged (greater than 0.20 second) but constant
- QRS: Usually 0.10 second or less in duration

Rhythm Recognition

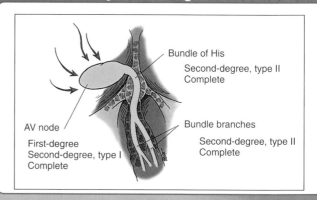

Bundle of His
Second-degree, type II
Complete

AV node

First-degree
Second-degree, type I
Complete

Bundle branches
Second-degree, type II
Complete

Rhythm Recognition

100% paced rhythm—AV sequential pacemaker
- Atrial paced activity? Yes
- Ventricular paced activity? Yes
- Paced interval rate? 88

Rhythm Recognition

A rhythm that is ventricular in origin has an intrinsic rate of 20 to 40 beats/min and is called a(n) idioventricular rhythm (IVR) or ventricular escape rhythm.

If the ventricular rate increases to a rate of 40 to 100 beats/min the rhythm is called a(n) accelerated idioventricular rhythm (AIVR).

If the ventricular rate exceeds 100 beats/min it is called ventricular tachycardia.

Rhythm Recognition

This rhythm strip is from a 69-year-old man complaining of shortness of breath. Lung sounds reveal bilateral crackles. Blood pressure 160/58. Identify the rhythm (lead II).

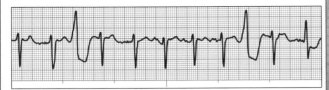

Rhythm Recognition

This rhythm strip is from a 90-year-old woman complaining of difficulty breathing. Identify the rhythm (lead II).

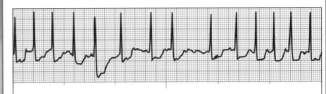

Rhythm Recognition

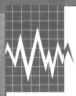

Describe the appearance of second-degree AV block, 2:1 conduction on the cardiac monitor.

Rhythm Recognition

Identify the rhythm.

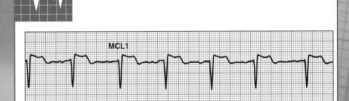

MCL1

Rhythm Recognition

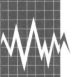

This rhythm strip is from a 59-year-old woman complaining of chest pain. She has a history of congestive heart failure and seizures. Identify the rhythm (lead II).

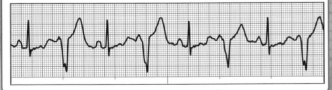

Rhythm Recognition

Identify the rhythm.

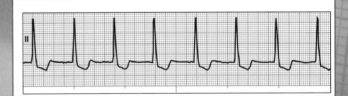

Rhythm Recognition

This rhythm strip is from a 17-year-old male who experienced a syncopal episode while playing baseball in 110°F heat for 4 hours. Blood pressure 148/84. Core temperature 101.8°F. Identify the rhythm (lead II).

The cardiac monitor shows a wide-QRS tachycardia. Name three possible origins of this rhythm.

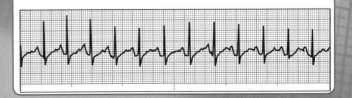

Rhythm Recognition

Atrial fibrillation (uncontrolled)
- Ventricular rhythm: Irregular
- Ventricular rate: 83 to 167/min
- Atrial rhythm: Unable to determine
- Atrial rate: Unable to determine
- PRI: Unable to determine
- QRS: 0.06 to 0.08 second

Rhythm Recognition

Sinus tachycardia with uniform PVCs
- Ventricular rhythm: Regular except for the events
- Ventricular rate: 107/min (sinus beats)
- Atrial rhythm: Regular except for the events
- Atrial rate: 107/min (sinus beats)
- PRI: 0.20 second (sinus beats)
- QRS: 0.08 second (sinus beats)

Rhythm Recognition

Sinus rhythm with first-degree AV block, ST-segment elevation
- Ventricular rhythm: Regular
- Ventricular rate: 68/min
- Atrial rhythm: Regular
- Atrial rate: 68/min
- PRI: 0.24 second
- QRS: 0.06 to 0.08 second

Rhythm Recognition

Second-degree AV block, 2:1 conduction:
- More P waves than QRS complexes
- P waves occur regularly
- Every other P wave is followed by a QRS
- The PR interval is constant
- The QRS may be wide or narrow
  - Narrow if the block occurs above the bundle of His (probably second-degree AV block, type I)
  - Wide if the block occurs at or below the bundle of His (probably second-degree AV block, type II)

Rhythm Recognition

Accelerated junctional rhythm
- Ventricular rhythm: Regular
- Ventricular rate: 75/min
- Atrial rhythm: None
- Atrial rate: None
- PRI: None
- QRS: 0.08 second

Rhythm Recognition

Sinus bradycardia with ventricular bigeminy
- Ventricular rhythm: Regular except for the event
- Ventricular rate: 39/min (sinus beats)
- Atrial rhythm: Regular except for the event
- Atrial rate: 39/min (sinus beats)
- PRI: 0.20 second (sinus beats)
- QRS: 0.08 second (sinus beats)

Rhythm Recognition

Sinus tachycardia
- Ventricular rhythm: Regular
- Ventricular rate: 125/min
- Atrial rhythm: Regular
- Atrial rate: 125/min
- PRI: 0.16 second
- QRS: 0.06 second

Rhythm Recognition

Possible origins of a wide-QRS tachycardia include the following:
- Ventricular tachycardia
- Supraventricular tachycardia with aberrant conduction
- Supraventricular tachycardia with an underlying bundle branch block
- Wolff-Parkinson-White syndrome

Rhythm Recognition

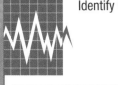

Identify the rhythm (lead II).

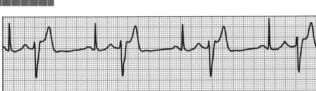

ORS   PR lengthen   QRS

Rhythm Recognition

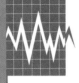

This rhythm strip is from a 79-year-old woman with epistaxis. Blood pressure = 222/118. Identify the rhythm (lead II).

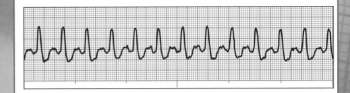

Rhythm Recognition

Identify the rhythm (lead II).

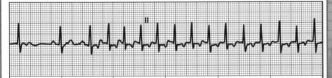

Rhythm Recognition

Identify the rhythm (lead II).

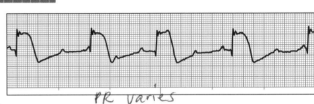

PR varies

Rhythm Recognition

A 43-year-old woman is complaining of palpitations. The patient has a history of SVT and states that she cannot tolerate adenosine. The following rhythm is observed on the cardiac monitor after diltiazem administration. Identify the rhythm.

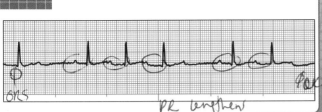

Rhythm Recognition

Identify the rhythm (lead II).

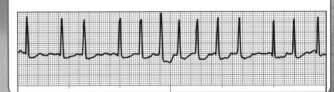

Rhythm Recognition

This rhythm strip is from an 18-year-old man with a gunshot wound to his chest. Identify the rhythm (lead II).

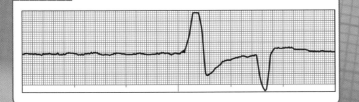

Rhythm Recognition

Identify the rhythm.

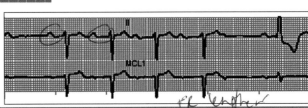

PR lengthen

Rhythm Recognition

Sinus tachycardia with a wide-QRS and ST-segment depression
- Ventricular rhythm: Regular
- Ventricular rate: 130/min
- Atrial rhythm: Regular
- Atrial rate: 130/min
- PRI: 0.16 second
- QRS: 0.12 second

Rhythm Recognition

Second-degree AV block type 1
- Ventricular rhythm: Irregular
- Ventricular rate: 51 to 83/min
- Atrial rhythm: Regular
- Atrial rate: 88/min
- PRI: Lengthens
- QRS: 0.06 second

Rhythm Recognition

Complete (third-degree) AV block with ST-segment elevation
- Ventricular rhythm: Regular
- Ventricular rate: 47/min
- Atrial rhythm: Regular
- Atrial rate: 115/min
- PRI: Varies
- QRS: 0.08 second

Rhythm Recognition

Sinus bradycardia with ventricular bigeminy
- Ventricular rhythm: Regular except for the event (every other beat is an ectopic beat)
- Ventricular rate: 36/min (sinus beats)
- Atrial rhythm: Regular except for the event
- Atrial rate: 36/min (sinus beats)
- PRI: 0.16 to 0.18 second (sinus beats)
- QRS: 0.04 to 0.06 second (sinus beats)

Rhythm Recognition

Atrial fibrillation
- Ventricular rhythm: Irregular
- Ventricular rate: 88 to 167/min
- Atrial rhythm: Unable to determine
- Atrial rate: Unable to determine
- PRI: Unable to determine
- QRS: 0.06 to 0.08 second

Rhythm Recognition

Junctional to sinus to narrow-QRS tachycardia
- Ventricular rhythm: Regular (atrial beats)
- Ventricular rate: 187/min (atrial beats)
- Atrial rhythm: Unable to determine
- Atrial rate: Unable to determine
- PRI: Unable to determine
- QRS: 0.08 second (atrial beats)

Rhythm Recognition

Second-degree AV block, type 1 with a ventricular complex
- Ventricular rhythm: Regular
- Ventricular rate: 42 to 68/min
- Atrial rhythm: Regular
- Atrial rate: 68/min
- PRI: Lengthens
- QRS: 0.10 second

Rhythm Recognition

Agonal rhythm/asystole
- Ventricular rhythm: None
- Ventricular rate: None
- Atrial rhythm: None
- Atrial rate: None
- PRI: None
- QRS: 0.28 second

Rhythm Recognition

Identify the rhythm (lead II).

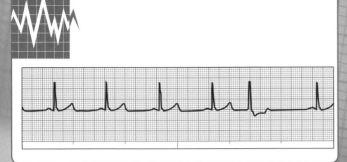

Rhythm Recognition

Identify the rhythm (lead II).

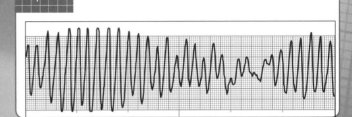

Rhythm Recognition

This rhythm strip is a 71-year-old man with abdominal pain. Identify the rhythm (lead II).

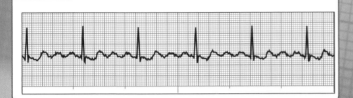

Rhythm Recognition

This rhythm strip is from a 27-year-old asymptomatic woman. Identify the rhythm (lead II).

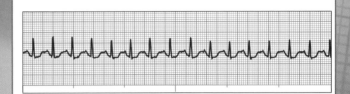

Rhythm Recognition

Identify the rhythm (lead II).

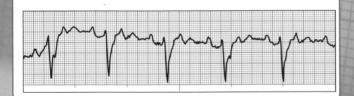

Rhythm Recognition

This rhythm strip is from a 61-year-old man found unresponsive, apneic, and pulseless. Identify the rhythm (lead II).

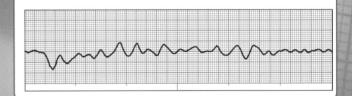

Rhythm Recognition

Identify the rhythm (lead II).

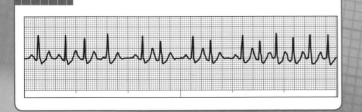

Rhythm Recognition

This rhythm strip is from a 19-year-old man after a seizure. Identify the rhythm (lead II).

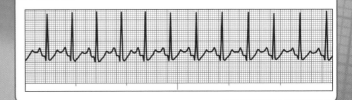

Rhythm Recognition

Polymorphic ventricular tachycardia
- Ventricular rhythm: Irregular
- Ventricular rate: 300 to 375/min
- Atrial rhythm: Unable to determine
- Atrial rate: Unable to determine
- PRI: Unable to determine
- QRS: Varies

Rhythm Recognition

Sinus rhythm with a PJC
- Ventricular rhythm: Regular except for the event
- Ventricular rate: 60/min (sinus beats)
- Atrial rhythm: Regular except for the event
- Atrial rate: 60/min (sinus beats)
- PRI: 0.14 second (sinus beats)
- QRS: 0.06 second

Rhythm Recognition

Sinus tachycardia
- Ventricular rhythm: Regular
- Ventricular rate: 157/min
- Atrial rhythm: Regular
- Atrial rate: 157/min
- PRI: 0.14 second
- QRS: 0.08 second

Rhythm Recognition

Atrial flutter
- Ventricular rhythm: Regular
- Ventricular rate: 55/min
- Atrial rhythm: Unable to determine
- Atrial rate: Unable to determine
- PRI: Unable to determine
- QRS: 0.08 second

Rhythm Recognition

Ventricular fibrillation (VF) (changing from coarse to fine VF)
- Ventricular rhythm: Unable to determine
- Ventricular rate: Unable to determine
- Atrial rhythm: Unable to determine
- Atrial rate: Unable to determine
- PRI: Unable to determine
- QRS: Unable to determine

Rhythm Recognition

Second-degree AV block, 2:1 conduction, probably type 2, with ST-segment depression
- Ventricular rhythm: Regular
- Ventricular rate: 54/min
- Atrial rhythm: Regular
- Atrial rate: 107/min
- PRI: 0.28 second
- QRS: 0.16 to 0.20 second

Rhythm Recognition

Sinus tachycardia
- Ventricular rhythm: Regular
- Ventricular rate: 120/min
- Atrial rhythm: Regular
- Atrial rate: 120/min
- PRI: 0.16 second
- QRS: 0.08 to 0.10 second

Rhythm Recognition

Sinus rhythm with PACs to narrow-QRS tachycardia
- Ventricular rhythm: Irregular to regular
- Ventricular rate: 63/min (sinus beats) to 188/min
- Atrial rhythm: Irregular to unable to determine
- Atrial rate: 63/min (sinus beats) to unable to determine
- PRI: 0.16 second (sinus beats) to unable to determine
- QRS: 0.06 second

Electrical Therapy

What is the purpose of defibrillation?

Electrical Therapy

Explain why it is important to look for and remove, if present, transdermal delivery patches from the patient's chest before using electrical therapy.

Electrical Therapy

Name at least two advantages of hands-free defibrillation.

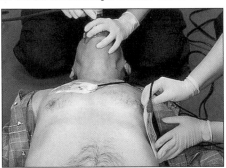

Electrical Therapy

What is an AED?

Electrical Therapy

State the correct energy settings for management of an unstable patient in atrial flutter with a rapid ventricular rate.

Electrical Therapy

Name three advantages of transcutaneous cardiac pacing.

Electrical Therapy

What is "synchronized cardioversion"?

Electrical Therapy

Name four possibilities to consider if the cardiac monitor displays a flat line.

Electrical Therapy

The aluminized backing used on some transdermal delivery systems can lead to electric arcing during defibrillation with the following:
- Explosive noises
- Smoke
- Visible arcing
- Patient burns
- Impaired delivery of current

Electrical Therapy

Defibrillation is the therapeutic delivery of unsynchronized (the delivery of energy has no relationship to the cardiac cycle) electrical current through the myocardium over a very brief period to terminate a cardiac dysrhythmia. The shock attempts to deliver a uniform electrical current of sufficient intensity to simultaneously depolarize ventricular cells, including fibrillating cells, causing momentary asystole. Defibrillation provides an opportunity for the heart's natural pacemakers to resume normal activity. The pacemaker with the highest degree of automaticity should then assume responsibility for pacing the heart.

Electrical Therapy

AED = Automated External Defibrillator

The AED is an external defibrillator with a cardiac rhythm analysis system that senses and records the rhythm and, if indicated, delivers an electrical shock. The shock is delivered by means of two adhesive pads applied to the patient's chest.

Electrical Therapy

- Enhances operator safety by physically separating the operator from the patient.
- May display less artifact than that shown on the ECG monitor when using hand-held paddles.
- Combination ("combo") pads allow ECG monitoring, defibrillation, cardioversion, and transcutaneous pacing through a single set of pads.

Electrical Therapy

Advantages of transcutaneous cardiac pacing include the following:
- Effective
- Safe
- Easy to apply
- Least invasive pacing technique available
- Can be used effectively by prehospital personnel, nurses, and other nonphysician providers with appropriate training

Electrical Therapy

If it is necessary to deliver an electrical shock to an unstable patient in atrial flutter with a rapid ventricular response, current recommendations include the use of synchronized cardioversion with energy levels of 50, 100, 200, 300, and 360 J (or equivalent biphasic energy).

Electrical Therapy

Possibilities include the following:
- No power
- Loose leads
- True asystole
- Isoelectric VF/VT
- No connection to the patient
- No connection to the defibrillator/monitor

Electrical Therapy

Synchronized cardioversion reduces the potential for delivery of energy during the vulnerable period of the T wave (relative refractory period). A synchronizing circuit allows the delivery of a shock to be "programmed." The machine searches for the highest (R wave deflection) or deepest (QS deflection) part of the QRS complex and delivers the shock a few milliseconds after this portion of the complex.

Electrical Therapy

Name two indications for defibrillation.

Electrical Therapy

What is the purpose of a vagal maneuver?

Electrical Therapy

Name two possible complications of transcutaneous pacing (TCP).

Electrical Therapy

You are preparing to defibrillate a patient in cardiac arrest. As you expose the patient's chest to apply the defibrillation pads, you observe a nitroglycerin patch on the patient's chest. How should you proceed?

Electrical Therapy

A 53-year-old woman is complaining of chest pain and begins losing consciousness. Her BP is now 50/P, and respirations are 12/min. The cardiac monitor displays a narrow-QRS tachycardia at 220 beats/min. Oxygen therapy was started and an IV was established before the patient's collapse. You promptly performed synchronized cardioversion with 50 J. Reassessment reveals that the patient is pulseless and apneic. The cardiac monitor reveals VF. What course of action should you take at this time?

Electrical Therapy

How does defibrillation differ from synchronized cardioversion?

Electrical Therapy

Management of unstable patients may necessitate the use of electrical therapy. Identify the correct energy settings for management of an unstable patient with atrial fibrillation.

Electrical Therapy

What is biphasic defibrillation?

Electrical Therapy

Vagal maneuvers stimulate baroreceptors located in the internal carotid arteries and aortic arch. Stimulation results in reflex stimulation of the vagus nerve and the release of acetylcholine. Acetylcholine slows conduction through the AV node, slowing the heart rate.

Electrical Therapy

Defibrillation is indicated for the following:
- Pulseless ventricular tachycardia (VT)
- Ventricular fibrillation (VF)
- Sustained polymorphic VT

Electrical Therapy

If a transdermal medication patch is present on the patient's chest, do not attempt to defibrillate through it. While wearing gloves, remove the patch and wipe the area clean before applying the defibrillation pads.

Electrical Therapy

Possible complications of TCP include the following:
- Coughing
- Skin burns
- Interference with sensing caused by muscle contractions or patient agitation
- Pain from electrical stimulation of the skin and muscles
- Failure to recognize pacemaker is not capturing
- Failure to recognize presence of underlying treatable VF
- Tissue damage, including third-degree burns, with improper or prolonged TCP
- Prolonged pacing has been associated with pacing threshold changes, leading to capture failure

Electrical Therapy

Defibrillation (unsynchronized countershock) has no relation to the cardiac cycle (a random discharge of energy).

Synchronized cardioversion uses a synchronizing circuit that allows the delivery of a shock to be "programmed" for a specific part of the cardiac cycle, thus reducing the potential for delivery of energy during the vulnerable period of the T wave (relative refractory period).

Electrical Therapy

If VF occurs during synchronized cardioversion, check the patient's pulse and rhythm (verify that all electrodes and cable connections are secure), turn off the sync control, and defibrillate.

Electrical Therapy

Defibrillators deliver current in "waveforms" that flow between two electrode patches (or paddles). For many years, defibrillators have used monophasic waveforms. Monophasic waveforms use current delivered in one (mono) direction through the patient's heart, from one electrode to the other. With biphasic waveforms, current is delivered in two (bi) phases—the current moves in one direction for a specified period, stops, and then passes through the heart a second time in the opposite direction.

Electrical Therapy

Current recommendations for the management of the unstable patient with atrial fibrillation are synchronized cardioversion with 100, 200, 300, and 360 J (or equivalent biphasic energy).

Electrical Therapy

Management of unstable patients may necessitate the use of electrical therapy. Identify the correct energy settings for management of an unstable patient with paroxysmal supraventricular tachycardia (PSVT).

Electrical Therapy

Describe four factors affecting transthoracic resistance.

Electrical Therapy

A 60-year-old man is complaining of dizziness that has been present for 3 hours. Oxygen is being administered and an IV has been established. The cardiac monitor reveals the rhythm below. The patient's blood pressure is 74/38, respiratory rate is 14. Breath sounds are clear.
What should be done now?

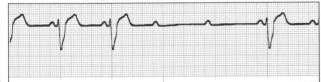

Electrical Therapy

A 54-year-old man is unresponsive, pulseless, and apneic. The patient weighs about 80 kilograms. The cardiac monitor reveals the following rhythm.
- You have a biphasic defibrillator available. Should the electrical therapy for this patient include synchronized cardioversion or defibrillation?
- What initial energy setting should be used in this situation?

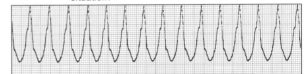

Electrical Therapy

What is transthoracic impedance?

Electrical Therapy

When using hand-held defibrillator paddles to deliver a shock, how much pressure should be applied to the paddles?

Electrical Therapy

Explain the difference(s) between manual defibrillation and automated external defibrillation.

Electrical Therapy

Name two advantages of the automated external defibrillator.

Electrical Therapy

Factors known to affect transthoracic resistance:
- Paddle/electrode size
- Paddle/electrode position
- Use of conductive material (when using hand-held paddles)
- Phase of patient's respiration
- Paddle pressure (when using hand-held paddles)
- Selected energy

Electrical Therapy

Current recommendations for the management of the unstable patient with paroxysmal supraventricular tachycardia (PSVT) are as follows: synchronized cardioversion with 50, 100, 200, 300, and 360 J (or equivalent biphasic energy).

Electrical Therapy

The rhythm shown is monomorphic ventricular tachycardia. Defibrillation is used to treat pulseless VT. When using a biphasic waveform defibrillator to treat pulseless VT/VF, use the energy levels recommended by the manufacturer for the initial and subsequent shocks. If you do not know what the recommended energy levels are, the 2005 resuscitation guidelines state that it is reasonable to use 200 J for the first shock. Use either an equal or higher dose for the second or subsequent shocks, depending on the capabilities of the device.

Electrical Therapy

The monitor shows second-degree AV block, type II. Preparations should be made for immediate transcutaneous pacing until a transvenous pacemaker can be inserted. A second-degree AV block, type II may progress rapidly to complete (third-degree) AV block without warning.

Electrical Therapy

When using hand-held defibrillator paddles, firm paddle-to-chest contact pressure (approximately 25 pounds) decreases transthoracic resistance by improving contact between the skin surface and the paddles and decreasing the amount of air in the lungs.

Electrical Therapy

Transthoracic impedance (also called transthoracic resistance) is the resistance of the chest wall to current flow.

Electrical Therapy

- Easy to use
- Reliable performance
- Permits remote, "hands-free" defibrillation
- Less training required to operate and maintain skills
- Speed of operation (delivery of first shock) faster than that with conventional defibrillators

Electrical Therapy

- Manual defibrillation refers to the placement of paddles or pads on a patient's chest, interpretation of the patient's cardiac rhythm by a trained health care professional, and the health care professional's decision to deliver a shock (if indicated).
- Automated external defibrillation refers to the placement of paddles or pads on a patient's chest and interpretation of the patient's cardiac rhythm by the defibrillator's computerized analysis system. Depending on the type of automated external defibrillator used, the machine will deliver a shock (if a shockable rhythm is detected) or instruct the operator to deliver a shock.

Vascular Access and Medications

Name three advantages of peripheral venipuncture.

Vascular Access and Medications

Name four local complications of intravenous therapy.

Vascular Access and Medications

Describe the effects of dopamine administration at 0.5 to 2 mcg/kg/min.

Vascular Access and Medications

Name three precautions that should be observed when administering sodium nitroprusside.

Vascular Access and Medications

A 75-year-old man has experienced a cardiac arrest. No intravenous (IV) line is in place. As the team leader of this resuscitation effort, indicate your sites of first choice in the placement of an IV line in this situation.

Vascular Access and Medications

Name three signs and symptoms of circulatory overload.

Vascular Access and Medications

How would you determine if an IV solution had infiltrated?

Vascular Access and Medications

Name a possible complication associated with the use of a catheter-through-the-needle device.

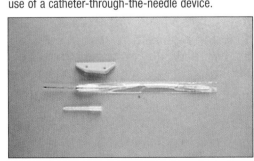

- Pain and irritation
- Hematoma formation
- Infiltration
- Extravasation
- Thrombosis and thrombophlebitis
- Venous spasm
- Vessel collapse
- Inadvertent arterial puncture
- Cellulitis
- Nerve, tendon, ligament, or limb damage

- Effective route for medications during cardiopulmonary resuscitation (CPR)
- Does not require interruption of CPR
- Easier to learn than central venous access
- If intravenous attempt unsuccessful, site is easily compressible to reduce bleeding
- Results in fewer complications than central venous access

- Can cause precipitous decreases in blood pressure. In patients not properly monitored, these decreases can lead to irreversible ischemic injuries or death.
- Monitor for signs of cyanide toxicity (disorientation, metabolic acidosis, nausea, muscle spasms, absent reflexes).
- Solution is sensitive to certain wavelengths of light, and must be protected from light during use. Wrap the IV bag in the aluminum foil package provided.
- Do not add other medications to this IV solution.
- Should be infused via an infusion pump.
- Sodium nitroprusside normally has a brownish tint when reconstituted. Discard the solution if it is strongly discolored.
- Use the solution within 4 hours of preparation.

At this dose range, dopaminergic receptors are stimulated, resulting in dilation of the renal, mesenteric, coronary, and intracerebral vascular beds. Diuresis usually occurs in this dose range and renal blood flow increases.

- Cough
- Crackles (rales)
- Chest pain
- Tachycardia
- Pulmonary edema
- Shortness of breath
- Distended neck veins
- Congestive heart failure

During circulatory collapse or cardiac arrest, the preferred vascular access site is the largest, most accessible vein that does not require the interruption of resuscitation efforts. If no IV is in place before the arrest, establish IV access using a peripheral vein—preferably the antecubital or external jugular vein.

When using a catheter-through-the-needle device, there is a risk of the sharp tip of the needle shearing off the end of the catheter, producing a catheter-fragment embolus.

Never pull backward through the needle. If you cannot advance the catheter through the needle, you must remove both the needle and the catheter.

One of the most reliable methods of evaluating infiltration is to apply a tourniquet above (proximal to) the infusion site tight enough to restrict venous flow. Infiltration is present if the IV solution continues to infuse despite the presence of the venous constricting band.

Backflow of blood into the IV tubing is not a reliable sign of patency of the IV line. The IV solution will seep into the tissues and flow into the vein if the catheter tip has punctured the wall of the vein. Other signs of infiltration include pain, pallor, or swelling of the IV site, a significant decrease in the infusion rate, coolness in the area of infiltration, or tissue sloughing.

Vascular Access and Medications

 Name five medications that can be given via the endotracheal route.

Vascular Access and Medications

 Give two examples of glycoprotein IIb/IIIa inhibitors.

Vascular Access and Medications

 Name two indications for administration of morphine sulfate.

Vascular Access and Medications

 When is lidocaine used?

Vascular Access and Medications

 An 82-year-old man has a blood pressure of 78/44. He experienced a massive anterior wall myocardial infarction (MI) yesterday and is now in cardiogenic shock. Dopamine is ordered for this patient. What is the rationale for this action?

Vascular Access and Medications

 Define inotrope.

Vascular Access and Medications

 Name two indications for verapamil administration.

Vascular Access and Medications

 Describe how you would manage a patient who suffered an air embolism as a result of IV therapy.

Vascular Access and Medications

- Abciximab (ReoPro)
- Eptifibatide (Integrilin)
- Tirofiban (Aggrastat)

Vascular Access and Medications

N = Naloxone
A = Atropine
V = Vasopressin
E = Epinephrine
L = Lidocaine

Vascular Access and Medications

Although amiodarone is the antiarrhythmic mentioned first in the pulseless VT/VF algorithm, lidocaine may be considered if amiodarone is not available.

Vascular Access and Medications

- Analgesic of choice for continuing ischemic chest discomfort unresponsive to nitrates
- Pulmonary vascular congestion complicating acute coronary syndromes (systolic blood pressure greater than 90 mm Hg)

Vascular Access and Medications

Inotrope refers to myocardial contractility. A positive inotropic effect refers to an increase in myocardial contractility. A negative inotropic effect refers to a decrease in myocardial contractility.

Vascular Access and Medications

Dopamine is the drug of choice for treatment of pump failure with a systolic blood pressure between 70 and 100 mm Hg. Dopamine administration should result in an increase in myocardial contractility and a subsequent increase in cardiac output.

Vascular Access and Medications

- Stop the IV infusion and check for air or leaks in the IV tubing.
- Turn the patient on his or her left side with the head down. This position may facilitate the movement of air to the right side of the heart and help minimize the movement of air into the arterial circulation.
- Administer high-flow oxygen.

Vascular Access and Medications

- Stable narrow-QRS tachycardia due to reentry if the rhythm persists despite vagal maneuvers or adenosine
- Stable narrow-QRS tachycardia due to automaticity (junctional, ectopic atrial, multifocal atrial tachycardia) if the rhythm persists despite vagal maneuvers or adenosine
- To control the ventricular rate in patients with atrial fibrillation or atrial flutter (*Note:* should not be given to patients with atrial fibrillation or atrial flutter associated with known preexcitation Wolff-Parkinson-White [WPW] syndrome)

Vascular Access and Medications

Name three indications for calcium chloride administration.

Vascular Access and Medications

Name four clinical indications of lidocaine toxicity.

Vascular Access and Medications

What is the recommended dosage range for morphine sulfate administration?

Vascular Access and Medications

What is the mechanism of action of glycoprotein IIb/IIIa inhibitors?

Vascular Access and Medications

For what cardiac arrest rhythms is it appropriate to use amiodarone?

Vascular Access and Medications

Describe the effects of atropine on the cardiac conduction system.

Vascular Access and Medications

Name at least four factors that should be considered when selecting an IV site.

Vascular Access and Medications

List two indications for intraosseous therapy.

Vascular Access and Medications

Indications of lidocaine toxicity are usually central nervous system related and include the following:
- Dizziness
- Drowsiness
- Mild agitation
- Hearing impairment
- Disorientation and confusion
- Muscle twitching
- Seizures
- Respiratory arrest

Vascular Access and Medications

- Known or suspected acute hyperkalemia
- Hypocalcemia
- Calcium channel blocker toxicity/overdose
- Pretreatment for calcium channel blocker administration
- Magnesium toxicity

Vascular Access and Medications

They prevent fibrinogen binding and platelet clumping.

Vascular Access and Medications

The recommended dosage range for morphine sulfate administration is 2 to 4 mg (give in 2 mg increments) via slow IV push; give additional doses of 2 to 8 mg IV at 5- to 15-minute intervals as needed.

Vascular Access and Medications

Atropine competes with acetylcholine at receptor sites, blocking the parasympathetic response (vagolytic action). Administration of atropine has the following effects:
- Increases heart rate (positive chronotropic effect) by accelerating SA node discharge rate and blocking vagus nerve
- Increases conduction velocity (positive dromotropic effect)
- Little or no effect on force of contraction (inotropic effect)
- *May* restore cardiac rhythm in asystole or bradycardic pulseless electrical activity

Vascular Access and Medications

- Pulseless ventricular tachycardia
- Ventricular fibrillation

Vascular Access and Medications

- Emergency administration of fluids and/or medications, especially in the setting of circulatory collapse where rapid vascular access is essential
- Difficult, delayed, or impossible IV access
- Burns or other injuries preventing venous access at other sites

Vascular Access and Medications

Factors to consider when selecting an IV site include the following:
- Purpose of the infusion
- Amount and type of IV fluid or medications to be infused
- Expected duration of IV therapy
- Accessibility of the vein
- Size and condition of the vein
- Patient's age, size, general condition, and preference
- Your experience and skill with venipuncture

Vascular Access and Medications

How is adenosine administered?

Vascular Access and Medications

Name three indications for IV cannulation.

Vascular Access and Medications

Explain the mechanism of action of calcium channel blockers.

Vascular Access and Medications

Describe the effects of dopamine administration at greater than 20 mcg/kg/min.

Vascular Access and Medications

Name four systemic complications of intravenous therapy.

Vascular Access and Medications

Describe two signs and symptoms of thrombophlebitis.

Vascular Access and Medications

Name three side effects associated with the use of nitrates.

Vascular Access and Medications

What is the recommended adult dose for medications that can be given via the endotracheal tube?

Vascular Access and Medications

Indications for IV cannulation include the following:
- Maintain hydration
- Restore fluid and electrolyte balance
- Provide fluids for resuscitation
- Administration of medications, blood and blood components, nutrient solutions
- Obtain venous blood specimens for laboratory analysis

Vascular Access and Medications

Because of its extremely short half-life (seconds), adenosine should be administered through a large-bore IV line as close to the heart as possible (such as the antecubital vein).

The initial bolus is 6 mg RAPID IV bolus over 1 to 3 seconds followed by a 20 mL saline flush. If no response, may repeat with 12 mg in 1 to 2 minutes. The 12 mg dose may be repeated once in 1 to 2 minutes.

Vascular Access and Medications

- Produces effects similar to norepinephrine
- Vasoconstriction may compromise the circulation of the limbs
- May increase heart rate and oxygen demand to undesirable limits

Vascular Access and Medications

Calcium channel blockers inhibit movement of calcium ions across cell membranes in the heart and vascular smooth muscle, resulting in the following:
- Depressant effect on the heart's contractile function (negative inotropic effect)
- Slowed conduction through the AV node (negative dromotropic effect)
- Dilation of coronary arteries and peripheral arterioles
- Decreased myocardial oxygen demand

Vascular Access and Medications

- A slowed or stopped infusion rate
- Aching or burning sensation at the infusion site
- Skin warm and red around the intravenous site
- Swelling of the extremity
- Throbbing pain in the limb

Vascular Access and Medications

- Sepsis
- Contamination and infection
- Hypersensitivity reactions
- Speed shock
- Emboli (pulmonary, catheter, air)

Vascular Access and Medications

The recommended dose of some drugs that can be given via the endotracheal route is generally 2 to 2.5 times the IV dose, although the optimal endotracheal dose of most drugs is unknown. For example, some studies have shown that the endotracheal dose of epinephrine should probably be between 3 and 10 times the currently recommended IV dose.

Vascular Access and Medications

- Hypotension
- Tachycardia
- Bradycardia
- Headache
- Palpitations
- Syncope

Vascular Access and Medications

Name three indications for central venous access.

Vascular Access and Medications

What is the primary neurotransmitter of the parasympathetic division of the autonomic nervous system?

Vascular Access and Medications

Explain why atropine may be used in cardiac arrest.

Vascular Access and Medications

When is the use of amiodarone indicated?

Vascular Access and Medications

Where is the external jugular vein located?

Vascular Access and Medications

Describe the mechanism of action of amiodarone.

Vascular Access and Medications

When should the dosage of lidocaine be reduced?

Vascular Access and Medications

Name three disadvantages of peripheral venipuncture.

Vascular Access and Medications

Acetylcholine is the primary neurotransmitter of the parasympathetic division of the autonomic nervous system.

Vascular Access and Medications

- Emergency access to venous circulation when peripheral sites are not readily available
- Need for long-term intravenous therapy
- Administration of a large volume of fluid
- Administration of hypertonic solutions, caustic medications, or parenteral feeding solutions
- Placement of transvenous pacemaker electrodes
- Placement of central venous pressure or right heart catheters

Vascular Access and Medications

- Pulseless VT/VF (after CPR, defibrillation, and a vasopressor)
- Polymorphic VT
- Wide-complex tachycardia of uncertain origin
- Stable VT when cardioversion is unsuccessful
- Adjunct to electrical cardioversion of SVT/PSVT, atrial tachycardia
- Pharmacologic conversion of atrial fibrillation
- Rate control of atrial fibrillation or atrial flutter when other therapies are ineffective

Vascular Access and Medications

Atropine is a parasympathetic blocker that can be considered in asystole and slow pulseless electrical activity. In cardiac arrest, it is possible that an absence of ventricular activity may be caused or worsened by excessive stimulation of the parasympathetic division of the autonomic nervous system. Since atropine blocks the effects of acetylcholine, it seems reasonable to administer atropine in these situations. Although anecdotal reports of the return of sinus rhythm after atropine exist, definitive evidence of its usefulness is lacking.

Vascular Access and Medications

- Slows conduction in the His-Purkinje system and in the accessory pathway of patients with Wolff-Parkinson-White (WPW) syndrome
- Inhibits alpha- and beta-receptors, and possesses both vagolytic and calcium-channel blocking properties
- Lengthens the action potential duration (and increases the refractory period) in all cardiac tissues, including the SA node, AV node, atrial cells, Purkinje fibers, and in the ventricular myocardium

Vascular Access and Medications

The external jugular vein lies superficially along the lateral portion of the neck. It extends from behind the angle of the jaw and passes downward across the sternocleidomastoid muscle and under the middle of the clavicle to join the subclavian vein.

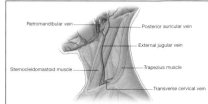

Vascular Access and Medications

- In circulatory collapse, vein may be absent.
- Phlebitis is common with saphenous vein use.
- Should be used only for administration of isotonic solutions. (Hypertonic or irritating solutions may cause pain and phlebitis.)
- In cardiac arrest, medications administered from a peripheral vein require 1 to 2 minutes to reach the central circulation.

Vascular Access and Medications

The maintenance IV infusion dose of lidocaine is 1 to 4 mg/min. This should be reduced after 24 hours (to 1 to 2 mg/min) or in the setting of altered metabolism (congestive heart failure, hepatic dysfunction, acute myocardial infarction [MI] with hypotension or shock, patients who are older than 70 years of age, poor peripheral perfusion), and as guided by blood level monitoring.

Vascular Access and Medications

Name the adrenergic-receptor sites stimulated by epinephrine.

Vascular Access and Medications

Name three side effects of atropine administration.

Vascular Access and Medications

What is the recommended dosage range for verapamil administration?

Vascular Access and Medications

Define chronotrope.

Vascular Access and Medications

Name the primary target organs affected by stimulation of the following receptor sites:
- Alpha-1
- Beta-1
- Beta-2

Vascular Access and Medications

Which of the following medications stimulate alpha-adrenergic receptors?
Dopamine
Dobutamine
Furosemide
Epinephrine

Vascular Access and Medications

Describe the mechanism of action of sodium nitroprusside.

Vascular Access and Medications

Name four signs and symptoms of digitalis toxicity.

- Cardiovascular:
  - Palpitations, tachycardia, possible extension of myocardial infarction (MI), angina, ventricular ectopy
- Central nervous system (CNS):
  - Anxiety, dizziness, headache, confusion, delirium
- Other:
  - Blurred vision, pupil dilation
  - Dry mouth, acute urine retention
  - Decreased sweating, flushed skin

Epinephrine stimulates alpha- and beta-adrenergic receptor sites.

Chronotrope refers to heart rate. A positive chronotropic effect refers to an increase in heart rate. A negative chronotropic effect refers to a decrease in heart rate.

The recommended dosage range for verapamil administration is 2.5 to 5.0 mg slow IV bolus over 2 minutes (administer over 3 to 4 minutes in the elderly or if the patient's blood pressure [BP] is within the lower range of normal). May repeat with 5 to 10 mg in 30 minutes (if no response and BP remains normal or elevated).

Dopamine is a dopaminergic, alpha- and beta-adrenergic stimulator. Dobutamine stimulates alpha, beta-1, and beta-2 receptors.

Furosemide is a loop diuretic.

- Alpha-1 receptor sites are found in the eyes, blood vessels, bladder, and male reproductive organs.
- Beta-1 (one heart) receptor sites are located in the heart and kidneys.
- Beta-2 (two lungs) receptor sites are found in the arterioles of the heart, lungs, and skeletal muscle.

- Cardiac dysrhythmias
- Fatigue
- Weakness
- Loss of appetite
- Abdominal discomfort
- Psychologic complaints
- Dizziness
- Abnormal dreams
- Headache
- Diarrhea
- Nausea/vomiting
- Visual disturbances, including distorted yellow, red, and green color perception; blurred vision; and halos around solid objects

Sodium nitroprusside (Nipride) is a potent, rapid-acting peripheral vasodilator (arterial and venous). It has the following effects:
- Increases cardiac output
- Decreases preload and afterload
- Decreases myocardial oxygen requirements

Vascular Access and Medications

Name three effects of parasympathetic nervous system stimulation.

Vascular Access and Medications

Describe the dosing schedule for administration of sublingual nitroglycerin.

Vascular Access and Medications

Which of the following exert a positive inotropic effect?
- Digitalis
- Verapamil
- Dobutamine
- Dopamine

Vascular Access and Medications

Which of the following are ventricular antiarrhythmics?
- Lidocaine
- Verapamil
- Dopamine
- Procainamide

Vascular Access and Medications

When should procainamide be discontinued?

Vascular Access and Medications

What is the usual dosage of IV Lasix?

Vascular Access and Medications

Name two indications for diltiazem administration.

Vascular Access and Medications

Describe the effects of digitalis on heart rate and myocardial contractility.

Vascular Access and Medications

One sublingual nitroglycerin tablet or spray may be administered every 5 minutes to a maximum of 3 doses. Monitor the patient's blood pressure closely before, during, and after administration of the drug.

Vascular Access and Medications

- Conservation of energy
- Decreased heart rate
- Increased secretion of saliva
- Bronchoconstriction
- Increased peristalsis
- Increased gastrointestinal secretions

Vascular Access and Medications

Ventricular antiarrhythmics include lidocaine and procainamide. Verapamil is a calcium channel blocker used in the treatment of narrow-QRS tachycardias due to reentry or automaticity, and to control the ventricular rate in patients with atrial fibrillation or atrial flutter with a rapid ventricular response. Dopamine is a vasopressor used in the treatment of hemodynamically significant hypotension (in the absence of hypovolemia).

Vascular Access and Medications

Digitalis, dobutamine, and dopamine strengthen or increase the force of myocardial contraction (positive inotropic effect). Verapamil, a calcium channel blocker, exerts a negative inotropic effect (weakens or decreases the force of myocardial contraction).

Vascular Access and Medications

The usual dose of Lasix (furosemide) is 0.5 to 1.0 mg/kg IV bolus. Use less than 0.5 mg/kg for new-onset acute pulmonary edema without hypovolemia. Use 1 mg/kg for acute or chronic volume overload, as well as renal insufficiency.

Vascular Access and Medications

Endpoints for procainamide administration include the onset of hypotension, suppression of the dysrhythmia, widening of the QRS by more than 50% of its original width, and administration of a maximum total dose of 17 mg/kg.

Vascular Access and Medications

Digitalis has the following effects on heart rate and myocardial contractility:
- Slows heart rate (negative chronotrope)
- Increases myocardial contractility (positive inotrope)

Vascular Access and Medications

Diltiazem is a calcium channel blocker that may be used to control the ventricular rate in stable narrow-QRS tachycardias or atrial fibrillation or atrial flutter with a rapid ventricular response if the rhythm persists despite vagal maneuvers or adenosine in patients with an adequate blood pressure.

Vascular Access and Medications

 Name three situations in which the use of beta-blockers should be avoided.

Vascular Access and Medications

 What is the initial and repeat dosing schedule for sodium bicarbonate administration?

Vascular Access and Medications

 When is administration of norepinephrine indicated?

Vascular Access and Medications

 Briefly explain how Angiotensin-Converting Enzyme (ACE) inhibitors work.

Vascular Access and Medications

 Name two indications for the use of aspirin.

Vascular Access and Medications

 Explain why dobutamine may be used in the management of a patient with pump failure.

Vascular Access and Medications

 Name four possible side effects of adenosine administration.

Vascular Access and Medications

 Describe the mechanism of action of beta-blockers.

Vascular Access and Medications

The initial dose of sodium bicarbonate is 1 mEq/kg. The repeat dosage is ½ the initial dose every 10 minutes thereafter.

Vascular Access and Medications

Beta-blockers should generally not be administered to patients with hypotension, bradycardia, congestive heart failure (CHF), second- or third-degree atrioventricular (AV) block, or a history of bronchospastic disease.

Vascular Access and Medications

In the body, the hormone angiotensin I is converted to angiotensin II (the active form of angiotensin) by the action of angiotensin-converting enzyme (ACE). Angiotensin II causes vasoconstriction (more potent than norepinephrine) and increased aldosterone secretion from the kidneys. Aldosterone causes the kidneys to retain salt and water and to excrete potassium, leading to an increase in blood volume and blood pressure. ACE inhibitors prevent the conversion of angiotensin I to angiotensin II. As a result, blood vessels relax, reducing the pressure the heart must pump against, and decreasing myocardial workload. By increasing renal blood flow, ACE inhibitors help rid the body of excess sodium and fluid accumulation.

Vascular Access and Medications

Norepinephrine (Levophed) is indicated in the following circumstances:
- Cardiogenic shock
- Severe hypotension (systolic blood pressure [BP] less than 70 mm Hg) not caused by hypovolemia

Vascular Access and Medications

Dobutamine stimulates alpha, beta-1, and beta-2 receptors. It has a potent inotropic effect (i.e., increased myocardial contractility, increased stroke volume, increased cardiac output), less of a chronotropic effect (i.e., heart rate), and minimal alpha effect (i.e., vasoconstriction).

Vascular Access and Medications

- Chest discomfort or other signs/symptoms suggestive of an acute coronary syndrome (unless hypersensitive to aspirin)
- Electrocardiogram (ECG) changes suggestive of acute myocardial infarction (MI)

Vascular Access and Medications

Beta-blockers:
- Slow sinus rate
- Depress AV conduction
- Reduce blood pressure
- Decrease myocardial oxygen consumption
- Reduce the incidence of dysrhythmias by decreasing catecholamine levels
- Reduce the risk of sudden death in patients with an acute coronary syndrome

Vascular Access and Medications

- Cardiovascular:
  - Facial flushing (common), chest pain (common), headache, sweating, palpitations, hypotension
- Respiratory:
  - Shortness of breath/dyspnea (common), chest pressure, hyperventilation
- Central nervous system:
  - Lightheadedness, dizziness, tingling in arms, numbness, apprehension, blurred vision, burning sensation, heaviness in arms, neck, and back pain
- Gastrointestinal:
  - Nausea, metallic taste, tightness in throat, pressure in groin

Vascular Access and Medications

Briefly explain why sodium bicarbonate is used in the management of hyperkalemia.

Vascular Access and Medications

You have been instructed to give vasopressin to a 67-year-old man in cardiac arrest. The cardiac monitor reveals ventricular fibrillation. An IV has been established. How will you administer this medication?

Vascular Access and Medications

Name three indications for the use of procainamide.

Vascular Access and Medications

Explain the mechanism of action of Lasix (furosemide).

Vascular Access and Medications

What is the typical starting dose of norepinephrine?

Vascular Access and Medications

Which of the following IV infusions are infused in mcg/kg/min?
- Epinephrine
- Dopamine
- Lidocaine
- Dobutamine
- Procainamide

Vascular Access and Medications

Does administration of verapamil or diltiazem affect myocardial contractility?

Vascular Access and Medications

What are the signs and symptoms of magnesium overdose? What is the antidote?

Vascular Access and Medications

Give a one-time dose of 40 units IV push.

Vascular Access and Medications

Sodium bicarbonate is used in hyperkalemia to decrease serum potassium levels by temporarily shifting potassium into the intracellular fluid.

Vascular Access and Medications

Furosemide (Lasix) inhibits reabsorption of sodium and chloride in the ascending limb of the loop of Henle, resulting in an increase in the urinary excretion of sodium, chloride, and water—profound diuresis.

Vascular Access and Medications

- Stable monomorphic VT in patients with no signs of heart failure
- Control of rapid ventricular rate in atrial fibrillation or atrial flutter in patients with no signs of heart failure
- Control of rapid ventricular rate in atrial fibrillation or atrial flutter in patients with known Wolff-Parkinson-White (WPW) syndrome and no signs of heart failure
- AV reentrant narrow-complex tachycardias such as reentry SVT if no response to vagal maneuvers and adenosine and if no signs of heart failure

Vascular Access and Medications

- Dopamine and dobutamine are infused as mcg/kg/min.
- Epinephrine is infused as mcg/min.
- Procainamide and lidocaine are infused as mg/min.

Vascular Access and Medications

The dose of norepinephrine is 0.5 to 1.0 mcg/min by continuous IV infusion titrated to improve blood pressure (up to 30 mcg/min). The usual dose range is 8 to 12 mcg/min.

Vascular Access and Medications

Signs and symptoms of magnesium overdose include the following:
- Hypotension
- Flushing, sweating
- Bradycardia, AV block
- Respiratory depression
- Drowsiness, decreasing level of consciousness
- Diminished reflexes or muscle weakness, flaccid paralysis

Antidote = calcium

Vascular Access and Medications

Yes. These medications are calcium channel blockers and are negative inotropes (they decrease the force of myocardial contraction).

Vascular Access and Medications

What is the usual dosage range for dobutamine administration?

Vascular Access and Medications

Name two potential advantages for the use of low-molecular-weight heparin (LMWH) over unfractionated heparin.

Vascular Access and Medications

Describe the mechanism of action of adenosine on the heart.

Vascular Access and Medications

You are instructed to administer diltiazem to a patient with a narrow-QRS tachycardia. How will you administer this medication?

Vascular Access and Medications

You are instructed to administer 80 mg of furosemide IV. At what rate should this medication be administered?

Vascular Access and Medications

Why are antiplatelet agents used in acute coronary syndromes?

Vascular Access and Medications

Name two advantages of external jugular vein cannulation.

Vascular Access and Medications

What are the preferred intravenous (IV) solutions for use in cardiac arrest?

Vascular Access and Medications

The advantages of using LMWH over unfractionated heparin include the following:
- Ease of administration
- Absence of need for anticoagulation monitoring
- Safety profile
- Potential for overall cost savings.

Vascular Access and Medications

The usual dosage range is 2 to 20 mcg/kg/min by IV infusion, but patient response varies.

Vascular Access and Medications

Initial dose 0.25 mg/kg IV bolus over 2 min. If needed, follow in 15 min with 0.35 mg/kg over 2 min. Subsequent IV bolus doses should be individualized for each patient.

Vascular Access and Medications

Adenosine is found naturally in all body cells and is rapidly metabolized. Adenosine has the following effects:
- Slows sinus rate
- Slows conduction time through AV node
- Can interrupt reentry pathways through AV node
- Can restore sinus rhythm in reentry SVT, including SVT associated with Wolff-Parkinson-White (WPW) syndrome

Vascular Access and Medications

Antiplatelet agents prevent thrombus formation by inhibiting platelet aggregation.

Vascular Access and Medications

Furosemide should be administered slowly IV push at a rate no faster than 20 mg/min. Ototoxicity and resulting transient deafness can occur with rapid administration. Do not exceed the recommended rate of infusion.

Vascular Access and Medications

The preferred IV solutions in cardiac arrest are normal saline and lactated Ringer's. Five percent dextrose in water is acceptable, but not preferred.

Vascular Access and Medications

The external jugular vein
- Is usually easy to cannulate
- Is considered a peripheral vein
- Provides rapid access to the central circulation

Vascular Access and Medications

What is the initial dose of amiodarone in cardiac arrest?

Vascular Access and Medications

Name three indications for the use of sodium bicarbonate.

Vascular Access and Medications

Describe the effects of dopamine administration at an infusion rate greater than 20 mcg/kg/min.

Vascular Access and Medications

When is the use of vasopressin indicated?

Vascular Access and Medications

Name four possible side effects of furosemide administration.

Vascular Access and Medications

Which of the following may be used in the management of both atrial and ventricular dysrhythmias?
- Verapamil
- Amiodarone
- Lidocaine
- Diltiazem
- Procainamide

Vascular Access and Medications

What is the recommended adult IV/IO dose of epinephrine in cardiac arrest?

Vascular Access and Medications

When is lidocaine contraindicated?

Vascular Access and Medications

- Known preexisting hyperkalemia
- Preexisting metabolic acidosis
- Specific overdoses, such as a tricyclic antidepressant overdose with QRS prolongation or hypotension

Vascular Access and Medications

Amiodarone is used in cardiac arrest due to pulseless VT/VF. The initial dose is 300 mg IV bolus. A repeat dose may be considered (150 mg IV bolus) every 3 to 5 minutes. If defibrillation is successful, follow with a 1 mg/min IV infusion for 6 hours. Then decrease the infusion rate to 0.5 mg/min IV infusion for 18 hours. Maximum daily dose is 2.2 g IV/24 hours.

Vascular Access and Medications

Vasopressin is used in cardiac arrest. However, at this time there is insufficient evidence to recommend for or against vasopressin use in pulseless electrical activity (PEA).

Vascular Access and Medications

At an infusion rate greater than 20 mcg/kg/min dopamine has the following effects:
- Produces effects similar to norepinephrine
- Vasoconstriction may compromise the circulation of the limbs
- May increase heart rate and oxygen demand to undesirable limits

Vascular Access and Medications

- Amiodarone and procainamide may be used in the management of atrial and ventricular dysrhythmias.
- Verapamil and diltiazem are calcium channel blockers used in the management of specific atrial dysrhythmias.
- Lidocaine is a ventricular antiarrhythmic.

Vascular Access and Medications

- Ototoxicity and resulting transient deafness can occur with rapid administration. Do not exceed the recommended rate of administration.
- Furosemide should be administered cautiously in patients with diabetes mellitus, dehydration, or severe renal disease.
- Patients with sulfonamide hypersensitivity or thiazide diuretic hypersensitivity may also be hypersensitive to furosemide.

Vascular Access and Medications

- Hypersensitivity to lidocaine or amide-type local anesthetics
- Severe degrees of sinoatrial, atrioventricular, or intraventricular block in the absence of an artificial pacemaker
- Stokes-Adams syndrome (sudden recurring episodes of loss of consciousness caused by transient interruption of cardiac output by incomplete or complete heart block)
- Wolff-Parkinson-White (WPW) syndrome

Vascular Access and Medications

The IV/IO dose of epinephrine in cardiac arrest is 1 mg every 3 to 5 minutes. There is no maximum dose.

Vascular Access and Medications

Cellulitis is one possible local complication of IV therapy. Describe the signs and symptoms of cellulitis.

Vascular Access and Medications

Name three indications for administration of adenosine.

Vascular Access and Medications

When is administration of naloxone indicated?

Vascular Access and Medications

Describe the mechanism of action of statins.

Vascular Access and Medications

Explain the mechanism of action of clopidogrel.

Vascular Access and Medications

When is sotalol indicated?

Vascular Access and Medications

List three examples of statins.

Vascular Access and Medications

When is sodium nitroprusside indicated?

- Stable, narrow-complex AV nodal or sinus nodal reentry tachycardias
- For unstable reentry SVT while preparations are made for cardioversion
- Undefined, stable, narrow-complex SVT as a combination therapeutic and diagnostic maneuver
- Stable, wide-complex tachycardias in patients with a recurrence of a known reentry pathway that has been previously defined

Cellulitis is a diffuse inflammation and infection of cellular and subcutaneous connective tissue that can lead to abscess formation and ulceration of deeper tissues. Signs and symptoms include pain, tenderness, warmth, edema, red streaking on skin (if spread to lymphatics), roughened appearance of the skin (like that of an orange peel), fever, and chills.

Statins have the following actions:
- Slow cholesterol production
- Lower low-density lipoprotein (LDL) cholesterol and triglyceride levels
- Increase high-density lipoprotein (HDL) cholesterol
- Increase the liver's ability to remove circulating LDL cholesterol

- Complete or partial reversal of narcotic depression, including respiratory depression, induced by opioids including natural and synthetic narcotics, propoxyphene, methadone, and the narcotic-antagonist analgesics: nalbuphine, pentazocine, and butorphanol
- Diagnosis of suspected acute opioid overdose

Indications for sotalol administration include the following:
- Monomorphic VT
- For rhythm control of atrial fibrillation or atrial flutter in patients with WPW syndrome if the rhythm has been present ≤48 hours and no signs of heart failure are present

Clopidogrel (Plavix) is an antiplatelet agent that helps prevent platelets from sticking together and forming clots. Platelets exposed to clopidogrel are affected for the remainder of their lifespan.

Sodium nitroprusside is indicated for the immediate reduction of blood pressure in a hypertensive emergency or hypertensive urgency.

Statins include atorvastatin (Lipitor); fluvastatin (Lescol); lovastatin (Mevacor); pravastatin (Pravachol); rosuvastatin (Crestor); and simvastatin (Zocor).

Acute Coronary Syndromes

What are acute coronary syndromes?

Acute Coronary Syndromes

Define myocardial infarction.

Acute Coronary Syndromes

What is the most common cause of an acute coronary syndrome?

Acute Coronary Syndromes

Name six terms patients may use to describe angina.

Acute Coronary Syndromes

A 70-year-old patient has chest discomfort. As you prepare to obtain a targeted history, your questions should focus on what areas?

Acute Coronary Syndromes

Which chamber of the heart is most often involved in acute myocardial infarction (MI)?

Acute Coronary Syndromes

What mnemonic is used to recall the interventions for most patients experiencing an acute coronary syndrome?

Acute Coronary Syndromes

Patients with acute coronary syndromes usually have chest discomfort, but they also may have atypical symptoms. Name three types of patients in whom atypical symptoms are most likely to occur.

Acute Coronary Syndromes

Myocardial infarction (MI) is myocardial cell death resulting from prolonged ischemia. In a practical sense, the term myocardial infarction is applied to the process that results in the death of myocardial tissue. Consider the "process" of myocardial infarction as a continuum rather than the presence of dead heart tissue. If efforts are made to recognize the process of myocardial infarction, patients may be identified earlier and, if promptly treated, may altogether avoid the loss of myocardial tissue.

Acute Coronary Syndromes

Acute coronary syndromes (ACSs) are conditions caused by a similar sequence of pathologic events—a temporary or permanent blockage of a coronary artery. This sequence of events results in conditions ranging from myocardial ischemia or injury to death (necrosis) of heart muscle.

Acute Coronary Syndromes

Common terms patients use to describe angina may include the following:
- "Heaviness"
- "Pressing"
- "Suffocating"
- "Squeezing"
- "Strangling"
- "Constricting"
- "Bursting"
- "Burning"
- "Grip-like"
- "A band across my chest"
- "A weight in the center of my chest"
- "A vise tightening around my chest"

Acute Coronary Syndromes

The most common cause of an acute coronary syndrome is decreased myocardial perfusion from coronary artery narrowing caused by a thrombus that has developed after plaque rupture or erosion.

Acute Coronary Syndromes

The left ventricle is the chamber of the heart most often involved in acute MI.

Acute Coronary Syndromes

The targeted history focuses on the following:
- The character of the pain
- Radiation, exacerbating or relieving factors
- Timing and nature of onset
- Risk factors for atherosclerotic heart disease
- Previous cardiovascular history

Acute Coronary Syndromes

Atypical symptoms are more likely to occur in patients with diabetes, women, elderly, nonwhite, and those with a high prevalence of congestive heart failure.

(Source: Pifarre R, Scanlon P, editors: Evidence-based management of the acute coronary syndrome, Philadelphia, 2001, Hanley & Belfus.)

Acute Coronary Syndromes

The mnemonic for the initial management of most patients with an acute coronary syndrome is MONA (morphine, oxygen, nitroglycerin, and aspirin). Generally, these agents can be administered within the first 10 minutes of patient contact (if there are no contraindications).

Acute Coronary Syndromes

Describe the electrocardiogram (ECG) changes seen in myocardial ischemia, injury, and infarction.

Acute Coronary Syndromes

Name the analgesic of choice for management of pain associated with ST-segment elevation myocardial infarction (STEMI).

Acute Coronary Syndromes

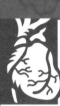

Name three signs and symptoms of pulmonary congestion.

Acute Coronary Syndromes

Define afterload.

Acute Coronary Syndromes

Describe the characteristics of unstable angina.

Acute Coronary Syndromes

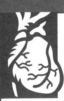

An inferior wall myocardial infarction is usually the result of occlusion of the _____ coronary artery.

Acute Coronary Syndromes

Name the "three I's" of an acute coronary event.

Acute Coronary Syndromes

Name four signs and symptoms of left ventricular failure.

Acute Coronary Syndromes

Morphine sulfate (2 to 4 mg IV with increments of 2 to 8 mg IV repeated at 5- to 15-minute intervals) is the analgesic of choice for management of pain associated with STEMI.

Acute Coronary Syndromes

- The zone of ischemia produces ST-segment depression or symmetrical T-wave inversion due to altered tissue repolarization.
- The zone of injury produces ST-segment elevation caused by abnormal repolarization.
- The zone of infarction (necrosis) may produce abnormal Q waves because of the lack of depolarization of necrotic tissue.

Acute Coronary Syndromes

Afterload is the force or resistance against which the heart must pump to eject blood.

Acute Coronary Syndromes

Signs and symptoms of pulmonary congestion may include the following:
- Dyspnea
- Cyanosis
- Tachypnea
- Frothy sputum
- Labored respirations
- Jugular venous distention

Acute Coronary Syndromes

An inferior wall myocardial infarction is usually the result of occlusion of the posterior descending branch of the <u>right</u> coronary artery.

Acute Coronary Syndromes

Unstable angina is characterized by one or more of the following:
- Symptoms that occur at rest (or minimal exertion) and usually lasting longer than 20 minutes
- Symptoms that are severe and/or of new onset (i.e., within the previous 4 to 6 weeks)
- Symptoms that are more severe, prolonged, or frequent in a patient with a history of stable angina
  Unlike stable angina, the discomfort associated with unstable angina may be described as painful. Patients with untreated unstable angina are at high risk of a heart attack or death. Early assessment and emergency care are essential to prevent worsening ischemia.

Acute Coronary Syndromes

- Pulmonary venous congestion/pulmonary edema
- Anxiety
- Orthopnea
- Cough with frothy sputum
- Tachypnea
- Diaphoresis
- Dyspnea

Acute Coronary Syndromes

- Ischemia
- Injury
- Infarction

Acute Coronary Syndromes

Name at least four common sites for anginal discomfort.

Acute Coronary Syndromes

Name three signs of cardiac tamponade.

Acute Coronary Syndromes

A 64-year-old man has chest pain. Name six possible causes that should be considered in the differential diagnosis of this patient's chest pain.

Acute Coronary Syndromes

Leads V_1 and V_2 view what area of the heart? What coronary artery typically supplies this area?

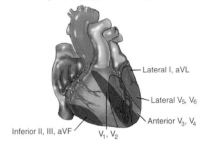

Lateral I, aVL
Lateral V_5, V_6
Anterior V_3, V_4
Inferior II, III, aVF
V_1, V_2

Acute Coronary Syndromes

Leads V_3 and V_4 view what area of the heart? What coronary artery typically supplies this area?

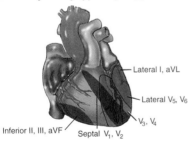

Lateral I, aVL
Lateral V_5, V_6
V_3, V_4
Inferior II, III, aVF
Septal V_1, V_2

Acute Coronary Syndromes

What associated complications may occur with a septal myocardial infarction?

Acute Coronary Syndromes

What associated complications may occur with an anterior wall myocardial infarction?

Acute Coronary Syndromes

A patient with a history of angina complains of ischemic chest pain of increased severity and duration. No ST-segment changes are observed on the 12-lead ECG. Describe how you will proceed to differentiate unstable angina from non–ST-segment elevation myocardial infarction (NSTEMI).

Acute Coronary Syndromes

Signs of cardiac tamponade include the following:
- Hypotension
- Pulsus paradoxus
- Distended neck veins
- Muffled heart sounds
- Narrowing pulse pressure

Acute Coronary Syndromes

Common sites for anginal pain include the upper part of the chest, beneath the sternum radiating to the neck and jaw, beneath the sternum radiating down the left arm, epigastric, epigastric radiating to the neck, jaw, and arms; neck and jaw; left shoulder; and intrascapular area.

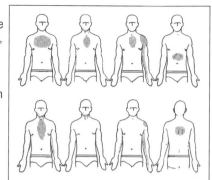

Acute Coronary Syndromes

Leads V_1 and V_2 view the septum. The coronary artery that supplies this area is the septal branch of the left anterior descending artery.

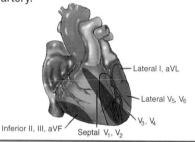

Lateral I, aVL
Lateral V5, V6
V3, V4
Inferior II, III, aVF
Septal V1, V2

Acute Coronary Syndromes

- Anaphylaxis
- Aortic dissection
- Cholecystitis
- Chronic obstructive pulmonary disease (COPD)
- Costochondritis
- Esophageal reflux, rupture, spasm
- Exercise angina
- Mitral valve prolapse
- Pancreatitis
- Pericarditis
- Pneumonia
- Pulmonary embolus
- Stress
- Anxiety
- Congestive heart failure (CHF)
- Herpes zoster
- Myocarditis
- Peptic ulcer
- Pleurisy
- Pneumothorax
- Pulmonary hypertension

Acute Coronary Syndromes

Associated complications of septal injury or infarction include possible bundle branch blocks or infranodal blocks because the area of damage often involves the septum, bundle of His, and/or bundle branches.

Acute Coronary Syndromes

Leads V_3 and V_4 view the anterior wall of the left ventricle. The coronary artery that supplies this area is the diagonal branch of the left anterior descending artery.

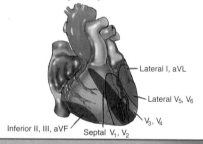

Lateral I, aVL
Lateral V5, V6
V3, V4
Inferior II, III, aVF
Septal V1, V2

Acute Coronary Syndromes

Patients with angina and no ST-segment elevation have unstable angina or NSTEMI. These conditions can be differentiated by the presence or absence of serum cardiac markers of myocardial necrosis. (Serum cardiac markers will be elevated in the presence of myocardial necrosis.)

Acute Coronary Syndromes

Associated complications of anterior wall injury or infarction include left ventricular dysfunction, congestive heart failure, bundle branch blocks, complete AV block, and/or ventricular dysrhythmias.

Acute Coronary Syndromes

Leads I, aVL, V$_5$, and V$_6$ view what area of the heart? What coronary artery typically supplies this area?

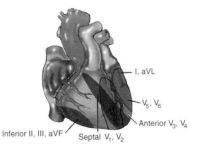

I, aVL

V$_5$, V$_6$

Anterior V$_3$, V$_4$

Inferior II, III, aVF   Septal V$_1$, V$_2$

Acute Coronary Syndromes

Define "definite" acute coronary syndrome.

Acute Coronary Syndromes

What associated complications may occur with a lateral wall myocardial infarction?

Acute Coronary Syndromes

Describe common signs and symptoms that may be experienced by an older adult having an acute myocardial infarction (MI).

Acute Coronary Syndromes

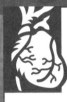

Explain how the use of beta-blockers may benefit the patient with ST-segment elevation myocardial infarction (STEMI).

Acute Coronary Syndromes

Describe the appearance of T waves in the early phase of a myocardial infarction.

Acute Coronary Syndromes

Name four possible complications of ST-segment elevation myocardial infarction (STEMI).

Acute Coronary Syndromes

A 59-year-old man has an ST-segment elevation myocardial infarction (STEMI). List four contraindications regarding the use of beta-blockers that must be considered in this situation.

Acute Coronary Syndromes

A definite acute coronary syndrome is a recent episode of typical ischemic discomfort that is either of new onset or severe or exhibits an accelerating pattern of previous stable angina (especially if it occurred at rest or within 2 weeks of previously documented MI). Triage is based on 12-lead ECG.

Acute Coronary Syndromes

Leads I, aVL, V$_5$, and V$_6$ view the lateral wall of the left ventricle. The coronary artery that supplies this area is the circumflex branch of the left coronary artery.

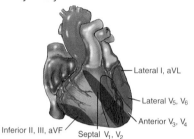

Lateral I, aVL

Lateral V$_5$, V$_6$

Anterior V$_3$, V$_4$

Inferior II, III, aVF   Septal V$_1$, V$_2$

Acute Coronary Syndromes

Chest pain typical of acute MI is described by only one third of patients more than 85 years of age. The most frequent symptoms of acute MI in older adults are shortness of breath, fatigue, and abdominal or epigastric discomfort. Older adults are more likely to have more severe preexisting conditions, such as hypertension, congestive heart failure, or previous acute MI; are likely to delay longer in seeking treatment as compared with younger patients; and are less likely to have ST-segment elevation on their initial ECG.

Acute Coronary Syndromes

Associated complications of lateral wall injury or infarction include left ventricular dysfunction and, in some patients, AV blocks.

Acute Coronary Syndromes

Although a myocardial infarction can produce changes in rate and rhythm, infarct recognition on the ECG relies on detecting changes in shape of the QRS complex, T wave, and ST segment. To review, one of the earliest changes that might be detected is the development of a tall (hyperacute) T wave. These T-wave changes may occur within the first few minutes of infarction, during what has been described as the hyperacute phase of infarction. These changes are often not recorded on the ECG because they have typically resolved by the time the patient seeks medical assistance.

Acute Coronary Syndromes

Several studies have shown the benefit of beta-blockers in STEMI. Beta-blockers
- Decrease heart rate, blood pressure, and myocardial contractility, resulting in decreased myocardial oxygen demand
- Lower early MI mortality
- Prevent malignant dysrhythmias, reinfarction, and myocardial rupture

Acute Coronary Syndromes

Beta-blockers should not be used if the patient has signs of heart failure, evidence of a low-output state, increased risk for cardiogenic shock (age greater than 70 years, systolic blood pressure less than 120 mm Hg, sinus tachycardia greater than 110 beats/min or heart rate less than 60 beats/min, and increased time since onset of symptoms of STEMI), or other relative contraindications to beta blockade (PR interval greater than 0.24 seconds, second- or third-degree AV block, active asthma, or reactive airway disease).

Acute Coronary Syndromes

- Pulmonary edema
- Dysrhythmias
- Papillary muscle dysfunction
- Right ventricular infarction
- Pericarditis
- Papillary muscle rupture
- Ventricular septal rupture
- Cardiac rupture

Acute Coronary Syndromes

Name three signs and symptoms of cardiogenic shock.

Acute Coronary Syndromes

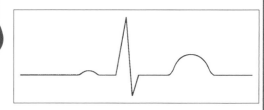

Locate the "J-point" on the illustration below.

Acute Coronary Syndromes

What types of dysrhythmias are particularly common with an inferior wall myocardial infarction (MI)?

Acute Coronary Syndromes

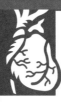

Define "possible" acute coronary syndrome.

Acute Coronary Syndromes

An 83-year-old woman in acute pulmonary edema has a blood pressure of 78/44. The cardiac monitor shows a sinus tachycardia at 110 beats/min. Describe your management of this patient.

Acute Coronary Syndromes

Tachycardia, jugular venous distention, dyspnea, diaphoresis, and dependent edema are signs and symptoms of _____ heart failure.

Acute Coronary Syndromes

A 72-year-old man is complaining of severe chest pain and weakness that has been present for approximately 3 hours. On a 0-to-10 scale, he rates his pain a 10. He is pale, he is diaphoretic, and his skin is cool to the touch. His blood pressure is 62/40. The cardiac monitor reveals a sinus rhythm at 90 beats/min without ectopy. Breath sounds are clear bilaterally. The patient has no significant past medical history and takes no medications regularly. How will you manage this patient?

Acute Coronary Syndromes

Explain what is meant by the term "contiguous leads."

Acute Coronary Syndromes

There is some difference of opinion as to where ST-segment deviation should be measured. Some authorities simply measure deviation at the J-point whereas others look for displacement 0.04 sec after the J-point. Still others measure ST-segment deviation 0.06 sec after the J-point.

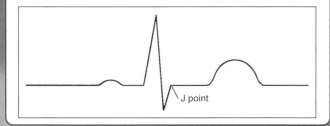

J point

Acute Coronary Syndromes

- Breathing may be labored, with audible coarse crackles or wheezing
- Marked tachycardia
- Cool and clammy extremities
- Poor peripheral pulses
- Varying degrees of end-organ dysfunction (e.g., altered mental status, decreased urinary output)
- Jugular venous distention may be present, suggesting right ventricular failure
- As ventricular dysfunction increases, pulmonary edema and severe hypotension may develop
- Restlessness, confusion, or unresponsiveness

Acute Coronary Syndromes

A possible acute coronary syndrome is defined as follows:
- Recent episode of chest discomfort at rest not entirely typical of ischemia but pain free at time of initial evaluation
- Normal or unchanged ECG
- No serum cardiac marker elevation

Acute Coronary Syndromes

Inferior wall MIs are frequently associated with the following:
- Sinus bradycardia
- First-degree AV block
- Second-degree AV block, type I (Wenckebach)
- Complete (third-degree) AV block with a junctional escape rhythm

Acute Coronary Syndromes

- Tachycardia
- Jugular venous distention
- Dyspnea
- Diaphoresis
- Dependent edema
- Fatigue (due to decreased cardiac output)

are signs and symptoms of right-sided heart failure.

Acute Coronary Syndromes

Initiate oxygen therapy, establish IV access, and prepare a dopamine infusion. Dopamine is the drug of choice for hypotension with a systolic blood pressure between 70 and 100 mm Hg that is not caused by hypovolemia.

Acute Coronary Syndromes

Electrocardiogram (ECG) changes are significant when they are seen in two contiguous leads. Two leads are contiguous if they look at the same area of the heart or if they are numerically consecutive chest leads.

Acute Coronary Syndromes

This patient is most likely experiencing an acute MI and is exhibiting signs and symptoms of cardiogenic shock. Give oxygen and establish IV access. Since there are no signs of pulmonary edema, consider a fluid challenge of 250 to 500 mL normal saline. If the response is inadequate, administer a norepinephrine infusion and titrate until the systolic BP (SBP) is 70 to 100 mm Hg. Once the SBP has increased to 70 to 100 mm Hg, attempt to switch to an infusion of dopamine.

Acute Coronary Syndromes

Cardiogenic shock may occur when approximately __% or more of the left ventricle is involved.

Acute Coronary Syndromes

A 75-year-old woman is exhibiting signs and symptoms consistent with acute pulmonary edema. She denies chest pain, but is severely dyspneic. Her blood pressure is 188/94, pulse is 144, respirations are 24 and labored. You are instructed to administered sublingual nitroglycerin to this patient. What is the rationale for this action?

Acute Coronary Syndromes

What is meant by the term "ejection fraction"?

Acute Coronary Syndromes

Explain the ECG criteria for significant ST-segment changes in a patient experiencing an acute coronary syndrome.

Acute Coronary Syndromes

Patients who experience a(n) _____ myocardial infarction (MI) have a greater incidence of congestive heart failure and cardiogenic shock than those who have MIs affecting other areas of the left ventricle.

Acute Coronary Syndromes

When is ST-segment elevation viewed on the ECG of a patient experiencing an acute coronary syndrome considered significant?

Acute Coronary Syndromes

How do you locate the TP-segment on an ECG and how is this information useful in a patient experiencing an acute coronary syndrome?

Acute Coronary Syndromes

Name four signs and symptoms of pulmonary edema.

Acute Coronary Syndromes

Nitroglycerin is administered to the patient with acute pulmonary edema (with a systolic BP greater than 100) to increase venous capacitance (promote venous pooling), thereby reducing preload (the amount of blood returning to the right atrium) and afterload (the resistance against which the heart must pump to eject blood).

Acute Coronary Syndromes

Cardiogenic shock is most often caused by extensive myocardial infarction. Because dead myocardium does not contract, when more than 40% of the ventricular muscle is involved, cardiogenic shock may result. Decreased contractility reduces the ejection fraction and cardiac output. This leads to increased ventricular filling pressures and dilation of the cardiac chambers. Systemic hypotension or pulmonary edema, or both, ultimately results from failure of one or both ventricles.

Acute Coronary Syndromes

ECG changes are significant when they are seen in two contiguous leads. ECG evidence of myocardial ischemia effects can be seen on the ECG as brief changes in ST segments and T waves in the leads facing the affected area of the ventricle. ECG evidence of myocardial injury in progress can be seen on the ECG as ST-segment elevation in the leads facing the affected area. In leads opposite the affected area, ST-segment depression (reciprocal changes) may be seen.

Acute Coronary Syndromes

Ejection fraction (EF) is the percentage of total ventricular volume ejected during each myocardial contraction. EF is used as a measure of ventricular function. Normally, the heart empties (ejects) slightly more than half the blood that it contains with each beat, thus a normal ejection fraction is more than 50%. Impaired ventricular function equals an ejection fraction of less than 40%.

Acute Coronary Syndromes

ST-segment elevation of more than 1 mm in two contiguous leads is the primary criterion used for infarct recognition. However, some cardiologists use a more stringent requirement for ST-segment elevation. In this alternate means of infarct recognition, at least 2 mm of ST-segment elevation is required in the chest leads before infarction is suspected. Each method has its advantage: The 1 mm threshold for ST-segment elevation favors sensitivity, and the 2 mm criteria favors specificity. Sensitivity refers to a test's ability to identify true disease. Specificity refers to a test that is correctly negative in the absence of disease. A test with high specificity has few false-positive results.

Acute Coronary Syndromes

Patients who experience an anterior MI have a greater incidence of congestive heart failure and cardiogenic shock than those who have MIs affecting other areas of the left ventricle.

Acute Coronary Syndromes

Signs and symptoms of acute pulmonary edema include the following:
- Tachycardia
- Diaphoresis
- Cough
- Foamy sputum
- Severe respiratory distress
- Severe agitation/confusion
- Crackles (rales), rhonchi, possible wheezes
- Hypertension or hypotension may be present
- Chest pain may or may not be present

Acute Coronary Syndromes

ST-segment displacement from the isoelectric line is used to detect myocardial ischemia and injury in a patient experiencing an acute coronary syndrome. Compare the ST-segment deviation to the isoelectric line. The TP segment is best used for this comparison; however, some authorities prefer to use the PR segment as the baseline.

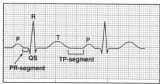

Acute Coronary Syndromes

Evaluation of a 12-lead ECG reveals marked ST-segment depression in leads V_1, V_2, V_3, and V_4. What do these ECG changes suggest?

Acute Coronary Syndromes

Explain the relationship between myocardial oxygen consumption and heart rate.

Acute Coronary Syndromes

A 65-year-old man is complaining of substernal chest discomfort that he rates a "7" on a scale of 0 to 10. His discomfort radiates to his left shoulder and jaw and has been present for about 4 hours. He is nauseated and diaphoretic. His blood pressure is 132/64 and his respiratory rate is 18. Breath sounds are clear. The cardiac monitor reveals the following rhythm in leads II, III, and aVF. Based on this information, are fibrinolytics recommended in this situation?

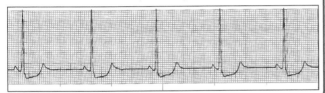

Acute Coronary Syndromes

What is Prinzmetal's angina?

Acute Coronary Syndromes

What is "ischemia"?

Acute Coronary Syndromes

What are the components of the "cardiovascular triad"?

Acute Coronary Syndromes

Why is tachycardia often associated with right-sided heart failure?

Acute Coronary Syndromes

What is the most common complication in the first few hours of acute myocardial infarction?

Acute Coronary Syndromes

Myocardial oxygen consumption is directly related to heart rate—the faster the ventricular rate, the greater the myocardial oxygen consumption.

Acute Coronary Syndromes

Marked ST-segment depression in leads V_1, V_2, V_3, and V_4 (reciprocal ECG changes) suggests posterior wall injury/ infarction. Reciprocal ECG changes are ECG changes in leads opposite the affected area.

Acute Coronary Syndromes

Prinzmetal's angina (also called Prinzmetal's variant angina or variant angina) is an uncommon form of angina. It is the result of intense spasm of a segment of a coronary artery. This variant angina may occur in otherwise healthy individuals (usually in their forties or fifties) with no demonstrable coronary heart disease. The episode of coronary artery spasm occurs almost exclusively at rest, often occurs in the early morning hours, and may awaken the patient from sleep. It is not usually brought on by physical exertion or emotional stress. Episodes usually last only a few minutes, but this may be long enough to produce serious dysrhythmias, including ventricular tachycardia and fibrillation, as well as sudden death. If the spasm persists, infarction may result.

Acute Coronary Syndromes

The rhythm shown is a sinus bradycardia with ST-segment *depression*. Fibrinolytics are generally not recommended for patients being treated more than 12 hours after symptom onset. They should not be given to patients being treated more than 24 hours after the onset of symptoms or to patients who show ST-segment depression (unless a true posterior MI is suspected).

Acute Coronary Syndromes

Cardiovascular triad:
- Conduction system (rate)
- Tank/vascular system (volume)
- Myocardium (pump)

Acute Coronary Syndromes

Ischemia is a decreased supply of oxygenated blood to a body part or organ. Myocardial ischemia can occur as a result of increased myocardial oxygen demand, reduced myocardial oxygen supply, or both. Angina is a symptom of myocardial ischemia.

Acute Coronary Syndromes

The most common complication in the first few hours of acute myocardial infarction is cardiac dysrhythmias, thus the reason ECG monitoring is essential.

Acute Coronary Syndromes

The body attempts to maintain cardiac output by increasing heart rate. The increased heart rate, however, results in decreased ventricular filling time.

Acute Coronary Syndromes

What is the "mirror test" and when might it be useful?

Acute Coronary Syndromes

How does myocardial injury differ from myocardial infarction?

Acute Coronary Syndromes

When should a right ventricular infarction (RVI) be suspected?

Acute Coronary Syndromes

A 62-year-old woman has signs and symptoms suggestive of an acute coronary syndrome. Her initial 12-lead ECG reveals nonspecific ST-/T-wave changes. What should be done now?

Acute Coronary Syndromes

Rearrange the following illustrations to correctly depict the typical pattern of ST-elevation myocardial infarction on the ECG.

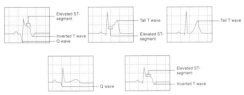
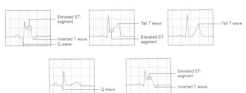

Acute Coronary Syndromes

Name two potentially lethal conditions that can mimic an acute myocardial infarction.

Acute Coronary Syndromes

Your patient is complaining of chest discomfort. Using the OPQRST memory aid, give examples of questions that should be asked of this patient.

Acute Coronary Syndromes

Name three conditions that can mimic myocardial infarction by producing ST-segment elevation on the ECG.

Acute Coronary Syndromes

Injured myocardial cells are still alive but will die (infarct) if the ischemia is not quickly corrected. If the blocked vessel can be quickly opened, restoring blood flow and oxygen to the injured area, no tissue death occurs. A myocardial infarction (MI) occurs when blood flow to the heart muscle stops or is suddenly decreased long enough to cause cell death.

Acute Coronary Syndromes

A posterior wall MI usually produces tall R waves and ST-segment depression in leads V_1, V_2, and to a lesser extent in lead V_3. To assist in the recognition of ECG changes suggesting a posterior wall MI, the "mirror test" is helpful. Flip over the 12-lead ECG to the blank side and turn it upside down. When held up to the light, the tall R waves become deep Q waves and ST-segment depression becomes ST-segment elevation—the "classic" indicative changes associated with MI.

Acute Coronary Syndromes

A normal ECG or nonspecific ST- and T-wave changes are nondiagnostic and require further evaluation. This patient is classified as intermediate/low-risk unstable angina. Obtain serial ECGs (ECGs every 5 to 10 minutes) and give aspirin and other therapy as appropriate (such as beta-blockers and nitroglycerin). Patients with a low likelihood of ischemia are initially managed in the Emergency Department Chest Pain Unit and then managed as outpatients with detailed evaluation within 72 hours.

Acute Coronary Syndromes

Suspect an RVI when ECG changes suggesting an inferior infarction (ST-segment elevation in leads II, III, and/or aVF) are seen. About 50% of patients with inferior infarction have some involvement of the right ventricle.

Acute Coronary Syndromes

Examples of potentially lethal conditions that mimic acute MI include aortic dissection, acute pericarditis, acute myocarditis, and pulmonary embolism.

Acute Coronary Syndromes

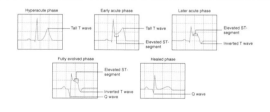

Acute Coronary Syndromes

Conditions that can mimic myocardial infarction by producing ST-segment elevation include left bundle branch block, ventricular rhythms, left ventricular hypertrophy, pericarditis, and early repolarization.

Acute Coronary Syndromes

OPQRST (pain presentation)	
Onset	"When did your symptoms begin?""Did your symptoms begin suddenly or gradually?"
Provocation/ Palliative	"Did anything bring on your discomfort?""Does anything make it better or worse?" (Associated with respiration, movement)
Quality	"How would you describe your discomfort?"
Region/ Radiation/ Referral	"Where is your discomfort?" (Ask the patient to point to it); "Does it go anywhere else?"
Severity	"On a scale of 0 to 10, with 0 being the least and 10 being the worst, what number would you assign your pain or discomfort?"
Timing	"Does your discomfort come and go, or is it constant?"

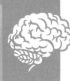

What causes an ischemic stroke?

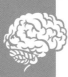

A 75-year-old man has signs and symptoms of a possible stroke. The onset of his symptoms began 45 minutes ago. Why is determining whether a stroke is ischemic or hemorrhagic an important step in determining therapeutic interventions for this patient?

An elderly patient is exhibiting signs and symptoms of a possible stroke. Her neck is auscultated for the presence of a carotid bruit. What is a bruit?

SLUDGE is a memory aid used to recall signs and symptoms of cholinergic syndrome. Explain what each of these letters represents.

What signs and symptoms are associated with significant beta-blocker toxicity?

Name three causes of wheezing other than asthma.

What signs and symptoms would you expect if a stroke affects the left side of the brain?

Your patient has sustained a gunshot wound to the chest. You hear a sucking sound from the wound each time the patient inhales. Describe how you will provide emergency care for the open chest wound.

Stroke and Special Resuscitation Situations

When a patient has signs and symptoms consistent with a possible stroke or transient ischemic attack (TIA), a computed tomography (CT) scan is frequently performed to rule out a hemorrhagic stroke, rather than confirm the presence of an ischemic stroke. This is essential if administration of a fibrinolytic (tPA) is being considered. Severe or even fatal complications may occur if fibrinolytics are inappropriately administered to a patient experiencing a hemorrhagic stroke.

Stroke and Special Resuscitation Situations

An ischemic stroke occurs when blood flow is blocked through an artery that supplies blood to the brain. This blockage may develop from a thrombus or an embolus. Thrombotic strokes occur when a blood clot develops within an artery supplying the brain (cerebral thrombosis).

Embolic strokes occur when a clot forms in another part of the body and then migrates to the brain (cerebral embolism). The clot often becomes lodged at bifurcations of arteries where blood flow is most turbulent. Fragments may become lodged in smaller vessels.

Stroke and Special Resuscitation Situations

- Salivation
- Lacrimation
- Urination
- Defecation
- Gastrointestinal distress
- Emesis

Additional symptoms include miosis (pinpoint pupils), bradycardia, bronchoconstriction, central nervous system depression, confusion, convulsions, seizures, and coma.

Stroke and Special Resuscitation Situations

A bruit is noise from turbulent blood flow that can be caused by narrowing of a vessel.

Stroke and Special Resuscitation Situations

- Pulmonary edema
- Chronic obstructive pulmonary disease
- Pneumonia
- Anaphylaxis
- Foreign bodies
- Pulmonary embolism
- Bronchiectasis
- Subglottic mass

Stroke and Special Resuscitation Situations

Signs and symptoms include the following:
- Bradycardia, heart blocks, and hypotension are the hallmarks of significant beta-blocker toxicity.
- Possible altered mental status; dyspnea due to bronchospasm or heart failure
- Possible bronchospasm in asthmatic individuals
- Seizures, coma, shock, cardiac arrest

Stroke and Special Resuscitation Situations

If a sucking chest wound is present, promptly cover the wound with an airtight dressing. Examples of dressings that may be used include plastic wrap, petroleum gauze, or a defibrillation pad. Tape the dressing on three sides (flutter-valve effect—the dressing is sucked over the wound as the patient inhales, preventing air from entering; the open end of the dressing allows air to escape as the patient exhales).

Stroke and Special Resuscitation Situations

A stroke on the left side of the brain will affect the right side of the body (and the left side of the face), producing some or all of the following:
- Loss of awareness or forgetting objects on the right side
- Weakness (hemiparesis), paralysis (hemiplegia), or lack of coordination of the face, arm, or leg on the right side of the body
- Lack of feeling and position on the right side of the body
- Difficulty speaking, listening, writing, reading, calculating with numbers, or understanding what others say (aphasia)
- Changes in behavior (slow, cautious)

Stroke and Special Resuscitation Situations

What is meant by the phrase "ischemic penumbra"?

Stroke and Special Resuscitation Situations

Name six signs and symptoms that may be associated with a tension pneumothorax.

Stroke and Special Resuscitation Situations

Poisons can be found in four forms. Name them.

Stroke and Special Resuscitation Situations

From what primary vessels does the brain derive its blood supply?

Stroke and Special Resuscitation Situations

What is the most common cause of hemorrhagic stroke?

Stroke and Special Resuscitation Situations

Give five examples of toxins that commonly cause seizures.

Stroke and Special Resuscitation Situations

Name the "four C's" of tricyclic antidepressant overdose.

Stroke and Special Resuscitation Situations

Name four common signs and symptoms of a stroke.

Signs and symptoms of tension pneumothorax include the following:
- Cool, clammy skin
- Increased pulse rate
- Cyanosis (a late sign)
- Jugular venous distention (may be absent if hypovolemia is present)
- Hypotension
- Severe respiratory distress
- Agitation, restlessness, anxiety
- Bulging of intercostal muscles on the affected side
- Decreased or absent breath sounds on the affected side
- Tracheal deviation toward the unaffected side (late sign)
- Possible subcutaneous emphysema in the face, neck, or chest wall
- Increased resistance felt during positive-pressure ventilation
- Falling O_2 saturation

In an ischemic stroke, there are two main areas of injury. The first area is the zone of ischemia. Because of the blockage in the artery, there is little blood flow through this area. As a result, brain tissue previously supplied by the blocked vessel is deprived of oxygen, glucose, and other essential nutrients. Unless blood flow is quickly restored, nerve cells and other supporting nervous system cells will be irreversibly damaged or die (infarct) within a few minutes of the blockage. The second area of injury is called the ischemic penumbra ("transitional zone"). The penumbra is a rim of brain tissue that surrounds the zone of ischemia. It is supplied with blood by collateral arteries that connect with branches of the blocked vessel. The size of the penumbra depends on the number and patency of the collateral arteries. Blood flow to brain tissue in this area is decreased (between 20% and 50% of normal), but not absent. Brain tissue in the penumbra is "stunned" but not yet irreversibly damaged. Because the collateral blood supply is not enough to maintain the brain's demand for oxygen and glucose indefinitely, brain cells in the penumbra may live or die depending on how quickly blood flow is restored in the early hours of a stroke.

The brain derives its arterial blood supply from the paired carotid and vertebral arteries and their branches.

Poisons can be found in four forms: solid, liquid, spray, or gas.

Toxins that commonly cause seizures include the following:
- Camphor
- Lithium
- Isoniazid
- Lidocaine
- Salicylates
- Beta-blockers
- Cocaine
- Tricyclic antidepressants
- Lead
- Phenothiazines
- Theophylline
- Amphetamines

The most common cause of a hemorrhagic stroke is high blood pressure. The constant force of high blood pressure weakens the walls of blood vessels, resulting in a brain hemorrhage.

- Sudden numbness or weakness of the face, arm, or leg, especially on one side of the body
- Sudden severe headache with no known cause
- Sudden dimness or loss of vision, particularly in one eye
- Sudden confusion, difficulty speaking, or trouble understanding speech
- Unexplained dizziness, unsteadiness, or sudden falls, especially with any of the other signs

The "four C's" of tricyclic antidepressant overdose are
- Coma
- Convulsions
- Conduction defects
- Contractility decrease

Stroke and Special Resuscitation Situations

Name three important abnormalities associated with asthma.

Stroke and Special Resuscitation Situations

Name six potentially life-threatening injuries that must be identified and for which treatment must begin in the secondary survey.

Stroke and Special Resuscitation Situations

What is a hemorrhagic stroke?

Stroke and Special Resuscitation Situations

Name four types of patients who are particularly at risk for hypothermia.

Stroke and Special Resuscitation Situations

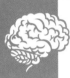

What toxin is associated with the odor of bitter almonds?

Stroke and Special Resuscitation Situations

Name six signs and symptoms of a hemothorax.

Stroke and Special Resuscitation Situations

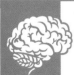

What is a transient ischemic attack (TIA)?

Stroke and Special Resuscitation Situations

Name four factors that determine the site and severity of an electrical injury.

Potentially life-threatening injuries that must be identified and for which treatment must begin in the secondary survey include the following:
• Pulmonary contusion
• Myocardial contusion
• Aortic injury
• Traumatic diaphragmatic tear/rupture
• Tracheobronchial disruption
• Esophageal injury

Asthma is a reversible obstructive airway disease characterized by three important abnormalities:
• Chronic airway inflammation
• Episodes of bronchoconstriction
• Mucous plugging

Neonates, trauma victims, intoxicated patients, the mentally ill, and the chronically disabled are particularly at risk for hypothermia.

A hemorrhagic stroke occurs as a result of rupture of an artery with bleeding onto the surface of the brain (subarachnoid hemorrhage) or bleeding into the brain (intracerebral hemorrhage).

Signs and symptoms of a hemothorax include the following:
• Tachypnea
• Dyspnea
• Hypotension
• Flat neck veins
• Pale, cool, moist skin
• Tachycardia
• Respiratory distress
• Narrowed pulse pressure
• Pleuritic chest pain
• Decreased breath sounds and dullness to percussion on the affected side with or without obvious respiratory distress

Cyanide

Factors that determine the site and severity of electrical injury include voltage, amperage, type of current (alternating versus direct current), resistance of tissues, current pathway, and duration of contact.

A TIA is a reversible episode of focal neurological dysfunction that typically lasts a few minutes to a few hours, resolving within 24 hours. During a TIA, an artery is temporarily blocked. A TIA is a significant indicator of stroke risk. About one fourth of patients with stroke have had a previous TIA. A TIA should be treated with the same urgency as a completed stroke.

Stroke and Special Resuscitation Situations

What is the most common cause of a subarachnoid hemorrhage?

Stroke and Special Resuscitation Situations

Name six assessment findings associated with anaphylaxis.

Stroke and Special Resuscitation Situations

Name four permanent neurological deficits that commonly result from a stroke.

Stroke and Special Resuscitation Situations

What signs and symptoms would you expect if a stroke affects the right side of the brain?

Stroke and Special Resuscitation Situations

Describe the basic life support modifications that should be made in the management of a pregnant patient in cardiac arrest.

Stroke and Special Resuscitation Situations

Name three major physiologic consequences of submersion.

Stroke and Special Resuscitation Situations

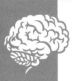

Current pathway is one factor that determines the site and severity of an electrical injury. Describe each of the following current pathways and indicate which is the most and least dangerous type of shock:
- Horizontal
- Straddle
- Vertical

Stroke and Special Resuscitation Situations

What factors determine the severity of a stroke?

Assessment findings associated with anaphylaxis include the following:
- Anxiety, restlessness
- Stridor, wheezing, coughing, hoarseness, intercostal and suprasternal retractions
- Tachycardia, hypotension, dysrhythmias
- Abdominal pain, vomiting, diarrhea
- Facial swelling and angioedema
- Urticaria (hives)
- Abdominal pain, cramping
- Pruritus (itching)

A cerebral aneurysm is the most common cause of a subarachnoid hemorrhage.

A stroke on the right side of the brain will affect the left side of the body (and the right side of the face), producing some or all of the following:
- Quick, impulsive behavior
- Difficulty drawing, dressing, or following a map
- Weakness (hemiparesis), paralysis (hemiplegia), or lack of coordination of the face, arm, or leg on the **left** side of the body
- Lack of feeling and position on the **left** side of the body
- Decreased ability to judge distances, size, position, rate of movement, and form
- Inability to think clearly
- Loss of awareness or forgetting objects on the **left** side of the body

- Problems with vision
- Weakness or paralysis
- Clumsiness or lack of balance
- Loss of sensation
- Difficulty with organization or perception
- Difficulty talking or understanding what is being said

The major physiologic consequences of submersion are hypoxia, acidosis, and pulmonary edema. Of these, hypoxia is the most important.

- The weight of the pregnant uterus on the inferior vena cava and aorta can hinder venous return and cardiac output (supine hypotension). To shift the weight of the uterus off of these major blood vessels, a patient who is 20 weeks pregnant or more should be placed 15 to 30 degrees back from the left lateral position. Maintain this position by placing a wedge, rolled blanket, or other object under the patient's right hip and lower back. If chest compressions are necessary, they should be performed with the patient in this position. Alternatively, the uterus can be manually displaced to the left.
- Chest compressions should be performed higher on the sternum (slightly above the center of the sternum).
- It is not necessary to modify energy settings or pad/paddle position if defibrillation is required.
- Before delivering a shock, remove fetal or uterine monitors (if present).

- The type of stroke
- The location of the obstruction
- How much brain tissue is affected
- How well the body repairs the blood supply to the brain
- How quickly other areas of brain tissue take over the work of the damaged cells

- In a horizontal (hand-to-hand or transthoracic) shock, current passes from one hand or arm across the chest and through the heart to the other hand or arm. Since the current passes through the heart, it is the most dangerous type of shock.
- In a vertical shock (hand-to-foot), the current passes from the hand and then down and out the lower leg or foot.
- In a straddle shock (foot-to-foot), current passes from one foot to the other. Because there are no major organs in the pathway of the current, this is the least dangerous type of shock.

Putting It All Together

A 75-year-old man is found unresponsive, pulseless, and apneic. The cardiac monitor reveals asystole. The patient was last seen 20 minutes ago. No history is available.

Name the medications (in order) that may be used in the management of this patient. Include the initial and repeat doses of each medication.

Putting It All Together

Name three possible causes of hypotension after a myocardial infarction.

Putting It All Together

How is amiodarone administered in cardiac arrest caused by pulseless ventricular tachycardia or ventricular fibrillation?

Putting It All Together

Name four dysrhythmias for which atropine may be used.

Putting It All Together

What is the preferred route for epinephrine administration in cardiac arrest?

Putting It All Together

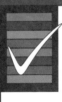

Name four therapeutic interventions that may be necessary for the patient with signs and symptoms of pump failure.

Putting It All Together

Name four rhythms for which vasopressin may be given.

Putting It All Together

Identify the correct energy settings for management of the unstable patient (with a pulse) in monomorphic ventricular tachycardia (VT).

Putting It All Together

- Rate problem (too slow or too fast)
- Volume problem (absolute or relative)
- Pump problem (decreased contractility)
- Vascular resistance problem

Putting It All Together

Epinephrine 1 mg (10 mL) of 1:10,000 solution IV/IO. May repeat 1 mg dose every 3 to 5 minutes *or* vasopressin 40 units IV × 1 in place of first or second dose of epinephrine.

Consider atropine 1 mg IV/IO repeated every 3 to 5 minutes to a maximum dose of 3 mg.

Putting It All Together

- Sinus bradycardia with hypoperfusion
- Symptomatic junctional escape rhythm
- Symptomatic second-degree AV block type I
- Symptomatic complete AV block at or above the level of the AV node (i.e., a narrow QRS complex)
- Asystole
- Bradycardic pulseless electrical activity

Putting It All Together

Initial bolus—300 mg IV/IO bolus. Consider repeat dose of 150 mg IV/IO bolus once in 5 minutes. If there is a return of spontaneous circulation, consider continuous IV infusion (1 mg/min infusion for 6 hours and then a 0.5 mg/min maintenance infusion over 18 hours). Maximum daily dose is 2.2 g IV/24 hours.

Putting It All Together

Patients in pump failure may require the following interventions:

- Treatment of a coexisting rate or volume problem
- Correction of underlying problems (e.g., hypoglycemia, hypoxia, drug overdose, poisoning)
- Support for the failing pump
- Agents to increase contractility (dopamine, dobutamine, etc.)
- Vasodilators to decrease afterload
- Vasodilators, diuretics to decrease preload
- Mechanical assistance (intraaortic balloon pump)
- Surgery (coronary artery bypass graft, valve, heart transplant)

Putting It All Together

Epinephrine should be given IV or IO in cardiac arrest. The IV/IO dose of epinephrine is 1 mg of 1:10,000 solution. Although it can be given endotracheally, some studies suggest that endotracheal epinephrine can produce a transient *decrease* in blood pressure. This effect is presumed to be due to beta$_2$-adrenergic receptor stimulation. This can cause hypotension and *lower* coronary artery perfusion pressure, which may lessen the potential for a return of spontaneous circulation.

Putting It All Together

Current recommendations for the unstable patient in monomorphic VT are synchronized cardioversion using 100, 200, 300, and 360 J (or equivalent biphasic energy).

Putting It All Together

Vasopressin may be used to replace the first or second dose of epinephrine in cardiac arrest. The four cardiac arrest rhythms are asystole, pulseless electrical activity (PEA), pulseless ventricular tachycardia (VT), and ventricular fibrillation (VF).

Putting It All Together

A 58-year-old man states, "My heart is racing." The cardiac monitor reveals a rhythm (in lead II) with the following characteristics:
- Regular ventricular rhythm
- Ventricular rate of 150 beats/min
- QRS complex that measures 0.10 sec in duration
- No definite sign of atrial activity

Name three possible origins of this cardiac rhythm.

Putting It All Together

Describe the proper technique for applying a "tourniquet" before peripheral intravenous cannulation.

Putting It All Together

A patient has signs and symptoms consistent with an acute coronary syndrome. A 12-lead electrocardiogram (ECG) has been obtained. A review of the 12-lead ECG is performed to categorize the patient into one of three groups. Name the groups.

Putting It All Together

Explain what is meant by the phrase "failure to pace." How would you recognize this pacemaker malfunction on a cardiac monitor?

Putting It All Together

A 73-year-old woman is complaining of palpitations. The cardiac monitor reveals monomorphic ventricular tachycardia.
If present, what signs and symptoms would suggest that this patient is hemodynamically unstable?

Putting It All Together

A 58-year-old woman has a blood pressure of 62/34, a pulse of 36, and a respiratory rate of 22 per minute. The cardiac monitor reveals a complete AV block with a wide QRS. You are instructed to administer epinephrine. Describe how you will administer this medication.

Putting It All Together

Describe the effects of dopamine administration at 2 to 10 mcg/kg/min.

Putting It All Together

Name three indications for the use of amiodarone.

Putting It All Together

The "tourniquet" (which is actually a venous constricting band) should be applied tightly enough to restrict venous blood flow without cutting off the arterial circulation. The tourniquet is too tight if a pulse cannot be palpated below the tourniquet site.

Putting It All Together

- Sinus tachycardia
- Paroxysmal supraventricular tachycardia
- AV nodal reentrant tachycardia (AVNRT)
- AV reentrant tachycardia (AVRT)
- Junctional tachycardia
- Atrial flutter with 2:1 conduction

Putting It All Together

Failure to pace is a pacemaker malfunction that occurs when the pacemaker fails to deliver an electrical stimulus or when it fails to deliver the correct number of electrical stimulations per minute. It is recognized on the ECG as an absence of pacemaker spikes (even though the patient's intrinsic rate is less than that of the pacemaker) and a return of the underlying rhythm for which the pacemaker was implanted.

Putting It All Together

Categorize the patient into one of three groups:
- ST-segment elevation or new or presumably new left bundle branch block (LBBB)
- ST-segment depression/transient ST-segment/T wave changes
- Normal or nondiagnostic ECG

Putting It All Together

In cases of symptomatic bradycardia, epinephrine is administered as a continuous IV infusion—*not* as an IV bolus. Administration of epinephrine by IV infusion permits careful adjustment of the dose administered according to the patient's clinical response. The dose of epinephrine by IV infusion is 2 to 10 mcg/min.

Putting It All Together

A patient is considered "hemodynamically unstable" if any of the following signs and/or symptoms are present:
- Chest pain
- Shortness of breath
- Altered level of responsiveness
- Low blood pressure
- Shock
- Pulmonary congestion
- Congestive heart failure
- Acute myocardial infarction

Putting It All Together

- Pulseless VT/VF (after CPR, defibrillation, and a vasopressor)
- Polymorphic VT
- Wide-complex tachycardia of uncertain origin
- Stable VT when cardioversion unsuccessful
- Adjunct to electrical cardioversion of SVT/PSVT, atrial tachycardia
- Pharmacologic conversion of atrial fibrillation
- Rate control of atrial fibrillation or atrial flutter when other therapies are ineffective

Putting It All Together

At this dose range, dopamine acts directly on the beta-1 receptors on the myocardium, resulting in improved myocardial contractility, increased SA rate, and enhanced impulse conduction in the heart.

Putting It All Together

Describe the immediate management of a patient in atrial fibrillation with a rapid ventricular response and signs of hemodynamic compromise.

Putting It All Together

Name four possible complications of transcutaneous pacing.

Putting It All Together

Name the components of the Cincinnati Prehospital Stroke Scale.

Putting It All Together

Name four indications for the use of amiodarone.

Putting It All Together

Name four cardiac arrest rhythms and indicate which are "shockable" rhythms and which are not.

Putting It All Together

Of the following, which are administered only by continuous intravenous infusion?
- Dopamine
- Atropine
- Epinephrine
- Lidocaine
- Dobutamine

Putting It All Together

Although many tasks in a cardiac arrest are important, name the four tasks that are most critical.

Putting It All Together

Describe the necessary steps to perform transcutaneous pacing.

Putting It All Together

- Coughing
- Skin burns
- Interference with sensing due to patient agitation or muscle contractions
- Pain from electrical stimulation of the skin and muscles
- Failure to recognize that the pacemaker is not capturing
- Failure to recognize the presence of underlying treatable ventricular fibrillation (VF)
- Tissue damage, including third-degree burns, has been reported in pediatric patients with improper or prolonged TCP
- Prolonged pacing has been associated with pacing threshold changes, leading to capture failure

Putting It All Together

If atrial fibrillation with a rapid ventricular rate results in hemodynamic compromise, immediate synchronized cardioversion is warranted with 100 J, and if the rhythm persists, 200 J, 300 J, and then 360 J (or equivalent biphasic energy).

Putting It All Together

- Pulseless VT/VF (after CPR, defibrillation, and a vasopressor)
- Polymorphic VT
- Wide-complex tachycardia of uncertain origin
- Stable VT when cardioversion unsuccessful
- Adjunct to electrical cardioversion of SVT/PSVT, atrial tachycardia
- Pharmacologic conversion of AFib
- Rate control of AFib or atrial flutter when other therapies ineffective

Putting It All Together

The Cincinnati Prehospital Stroke Scale consists of three parts:
- Facial droop (ask patient to show teeth and smile)
- Arm drift (ask patient to extend arms, palms down, with eyes closed)
- Speech (ask patient to say, "You can't teach an old dog new tricks" or similar phrase)

Putting It All Together

Dopamine and dobutamine are administered as continuous IV infusions, not as IV bolus medications. Atropine is administered as an IV bolus. Epinephrine is administered as an IV bolus in cardiac arrest, but as an IV infusion in symptomatic bradycardia. Lidocaine is administered first as an IV bolus and followed with a continuous IV infusion.

Putting It All Together

Shockable cardiac arrest rhythms include pulseless ventricular tachycardia and ventricular fibrillation. Asystole and pulseless electrical activity are cardiac arrest rhythms for which defibrillation is not indicated.

Putting It All Together

- Apply ECG electrodes
- Adjust cardiac monitor
- Apply pacing electrodes
- Select pacing rate
- Adjust output (milliAmps) until ECG shows electrical capture

Putting It All Together

- Airway management
- Chest compressions
- Monitoring and defibrillation
- Vascular access and medication administration

Putting It All Together

Name two indications for dopamine administration.

Putting It All Together

Explain why atropine should be used with caution in patients experiencing an acute myocardial infarction (MI).

Putting It All Together

Identify the rhythm below (lead II).

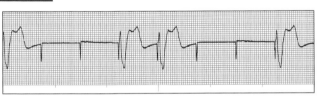

Putting It All Together

Name four dysrhythmias that may necessitate the use of synchronized cardioversion and the energy levels for each.

Putting It All Together

If an IV infusion is mixed with grams, it is infused in __.
   If an IV infusion is mixed with milligrams, it is infused in __.

Putting It All Together

Name four dysrhythmias that may necessitate the use of synchronized cardioversion and the energy levels for each.

A 65-year-old woman has been admitted to the coronary care unit with an ST-segment elevation myocardial infarction (STEMI). She indicates that she takes ibuprofen daily for arthritis pain. Should this medication be continued during her hospital stay?

Putting It All Together

What is the trade name for amiodarone?

Putting It All Together

Describe the ECG indicators of myocardial ischemia.

Putting It All Together

Atropine should be used with caution in acute MI because excessive increases in heart rate may further worsen ischemia or increase size of infarction.

Putting It All Together

- Symptomatic bradycardias that have not responded to atropine and/or when external pacing is unavailable or ineffective
- Hypotension that occurs after return of spontaneous circulation
- Hemodynamically significant hypotension in the absence of hypovolemia

Putting It All Together

- Paroxysmal supraventricular tachycardia (PSVT): 50, 100, 200, 300, 360 J (or equivalent biphasic energy)
- Atrial flutter with a rapid ventricular response: 50, 100, 200, 300, 360 J (or equivalent biphasic energy)
- Atrial fibrillation with a rapid ventricular response: 100, 200, 300, 360 J (or equivalent biphasic energy)
- Sustained monomorphic ventricular tachycardia: 100, 200, 300, 360 J (or equivalent biphasic energy)

Putting It All Together

The rhythm strip shown reflects a pacemaker's failure to capture.

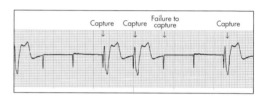

Putting It All Together

Nonsteroidal antiinflammatory drugs (except for aspirin) should not be administered during hospitalization for STEMI because of the increased risk of mortality, reinfarction, hypertension, heart failure, and myocardial rupture associated with their use.

Putting It All Together

If an IV infusion is mixed with grams, it is infused in milligrams.
   Example:
- Lidocaine infusion: 2 *grams* lidocaine mixed with 500 mL IV solution. Dose infused is 1 to 4 *milligrams*/min.
   If an IV infusion is mixed with milligrams, it is infused in micrograms.
   Example:
- Epinephrine infusion: 1 *milligram* epinephrine mixed with 250 mL IV solution. Dose infused is 2 to 10 *micrograms*/min.

Putting It All Together

ECG indicators of myocardial ischemia include ST-segment depression and T-wave inversion.

Putting It All Together

Cordarone

Putting It All Together

What is the usual dosage of dobutamine?

Putting It All Together

What is angina pectoris?

Putting It All Together

Describe the PR intervals for each of the following AV blocks:
- Second-degree AV block type I
- Second-degree AV block type II
- Complete (third-degree) AV block

Putting It All Together

A 58-year-old woman has chest pressure that has been increasing in intensity over the past 40 minutes. The patient has a history of angina. How is an MI distinguished from unstable angina?

Putting It All Together

Can atropine be used if a patient has a transplanted heart and is experiencing a symptomatic bradycardia?

Putting It All Together

Giving this drug too rapidly can cause tinnitus and transient deafness

Putting It All Together

When are glycoprotein IIb/IIIa inhibitors used in acute coronary syndromes?

Putting It All Together

Explain how administration of atropine to a patient with a symptomatic bradycardia and administration to a patient in cardiac arrest differ.

Putting It All Together

Angina pectoris is chest discomfort or other related symptoms caused by myocardial ischemia. If the process is not quickly reversed and blood flow restored, myocardial ischemia may lead to cellular injury and, ultimately, infarction. It is important to remember that angina is not a disease, but a symptom of myocardial ischemia.

Putting It All Together

Dobutamine is administered by continuous IV infusion. The usual dose is 2 to 20 mcg/kg/min IV, but patient response varies.

Putting It All Together

During their initial presentation, distinguishing patients with unstable angina from those with acute MI is often impossible because their clinical presentations and ECG findings may be identical. Early assessment, including a focused history, and intervention is essential to prevent worsening ischemia. Serial ECGs and continuous ECG monitoring should be performed. Serum cardiac markers should be obtained on initial presentation to rule out infarction and again in 6 hours.

Putting It All Together

- The PR intervals in a second-degree AV block type I (i.e., Wenckebach) progressively lengthens until a P wave appears without a QRS complex.
- The PR intervals in a second-degree AV block type II are constant before each conducted QRS complex.
- The PR intervals in a complete AV block vary because there is no relationship between atrial and ventricular activity.

Putting It All Together

Furosemide (Lasix)

Putting It All Together

Although transplanted hearts do not usually respond to atropine because they lack vagal nerve innervation, atropine may be used with caution after heart transplantation. Monitoring is essential.

Putting It All Together

When atropine is given to a patient experiencing a symptomatic bradycardia, the recommended dosage is 0.5 mg IV push every 3 to 5 minutes to a total dose of 3.0 mg. Do not push slowly or in smaller than recommended doses.

When atropine is given to a patient in cardiac arrest due to asystole/slow pulseless electrical activity (PEA), the IV/IO dose is 1.0 mg every 3 to 5 minutes to a total dose of 3 mg. The endotracheal dose is 2 to 2.5 times the IV/IO dose.

Putting It All Together

Glycoprotein IIb/IIIa inhibitors may be used in patients experiencing an acute MI without ST-segment elevation who have some high-risk features and/or refractory ischemia, provided they do not have a major contraindication because of bleeding.

Putting It All Together

It is 9:00 A.M. A 59-year-old man is complaining of weakness. The patient states that he vomited blood last evening at about 8:00 P.M. and then again this morning at 8:00 A.M. The patient states that he had episodes of rectal bleeding throughout the night. Initial vital signs are as follows: blood pressure 80/60, pulse 116 (weak, but regular), respirations 16 to 20. His skin is warm, dry, and pale. The cardiac monitor shows a sinus tachycardia.

Physical examination reveals that the patient's lungs are clear bilaterally. The abdomen is soft and the patient denies tenderness on palpation. The remainder of the physical examination is unremarkable. The patient has a history of duodenal ulcers, cirrhosis of the liver, and GI bleeding. His medications include Lasix and Lorazepam. How will you manage this patient?

Putting It All Together

What are three important questions to ask yourself when treating a tachycardia?

Putting It All Together

What is the inherent rate of the sinoatrial (SA) node?

Putting It All Together

Name two indications for the use of magnesium sulfate.

Putting It All Together

A 78-year-old man is anxious and complaining of palpitations. His vital signs are blood pressure 110/64, pulse 190, and respirations 16. The patient denies chest pain. Breath sounds are clear. The cardiac monitor shows monomorphic ventricular tachycardia. Is this patient stable or unstable? Describe your management of this patient.

Putting It All Together

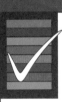

Describe the appearance of atrial activity in atrial fibrillation on the ECG.

Putting It All Together

A 64-year-old man is in cardiac arrest. The cardiac monitor reveals ventricular fibrillation that has not responded to an initial defibrillation attempt, administration of IV epinephrine, and a second shock. CPR is ongoing. What should be done next?

Putting It All Together

A 91-year-old man is in acute cardiogenic pulmonary edema. His blood pressure is 176/100. His respiratory rate is 38 and labored. The cardiac monitor reveals a sinus tachycardia. Name the first-line medications that may be useful in managing this patient.

Putting It All Together

Remember three important questions to ask yourself when treating a tachycardia.
- Is the patient stable or unstable?
- Is the QRS wide or narrow?
- Is the ventricular rhythm regular or irregular?

Putting It All Together

This patient is hypotensive. The key question to ask is: Are the patient's signs and symptoms due to a rate problem, a pump problem, a volume problem, or a vascular resistance problem? Given the patient's history of the present illness, we assume a volume problem exists.

Administer oxygen, establish two large-bore IVs of normal saline or lactated Ringer's solution, and administer a fluid challenge (a fluid challenge of 10 to 20 mL/kg may be ordered and the frequency of additional boluses adjusted depending on the patient's response).

Obtain pulse oximetry, 12-lead ECG, and chest x-ray.

Obtain laboratory studies, including CBC, electrolytes, blood type and cross, urinalysis, and ABGs.

Putting It All Together

- Polymorphic VT with prolonged QT interval (Torsades de Pointes)
- Rhythm control of atrial fibrillation ≤48 hours' duration

Putting It All Together

The inherent rate of the SA node is 60 to 100 beats/min.

Putting It All Together

In atrial fibrillation, the atria are not contracting, they are quivering. This produces an erratic, wavy baseline (fibrillatory waves, or f waves) on the ECG. P waves are not visible.

Putting It All Together

Based on the information presented, the patient appears to be stable. The drug of choice for a stable patient in monomorphic VT is amiodarone. Because the patient has a pulse, give amiodarone 150 mg IV over 10 minutes. Repeat as needed to a maximum dose of 2.2 g/24 hr. Alternative drugs include procainamide and sotalol.

Putting It All Together

First-line medications include the following:
- Oxygen
- Sublingual nitroglycerin
- IV furosemide (Lasix)
- IV morphine

Putting It All Together

If pulseless VT/VF continues despite CPR, two or three shocks, and giving a vasopressor, consider giving an antiarrhythmic. Amiodarone is an antiarrhythmic that blocks sodium channels, inhibits sympathetic stimulation, and blocks potassium channels, as well as calcium channels. In cardiac arrest due to pulseless VT/VF, the initial IV/IO bolus of amiodarone is 300 mg. If the rhythm persists, consider a repeat IV/IO bolus dose of 150 mg in 5 minutes. If there is a return of spontaneous circulation after giving amiodarone, a continuous infusion of the drug may be considered. Although amiodarone is the antiarrhythmic mentioned first in the pulseless VT/VF algorithm, lidocaine may be considered if amiodarone is not available.

Putting It All Together

 Name two components of the ECG that should be monitored closely during procainamide administration.

Putting It All Together

 Briefly describe the ways in which a patient with monomorphic ventricular tachycardia may have and the initial management of each.

Putting It All Together

 Describe correct anatomic placement for each of the chest leads (V_1, V_2, V_3, V_4, V_5, and V_6).

Putting It All Together

 Name four categories of dysrhythmias that may occur with a heart rate of less than 60 beats/min.

Putting It All Together

 A 35-year-old man is complaining of chest discomfort and difficulty breathing. He is disoriented and anxious. Examination reveals bibasilar crackles; a weak carotid pulse, and a blood pressure of 70/40. The cardiac monitor displays a regular narrow-QRS tachycardia at a rate of 220 beats/min. Is this patient stable or unstable? Describe your management of this patient.

Putting It All Together

 What is the typical starting dose of IV nitroglycerin?

Putting It All Together

 A 55-year-old woman is complaining of chest pain that radiates down her left arm. She rates her discomfort an "8" on a scale of 0 to 10. Her skin is pink, warm, and moist. Blood pressure is 144/80, and respiratory rate is 20/min. Lung sounds are clear. How will you manage this patient?

Putting It All Together

 A 68-year-old man was found unresponsive in his backyard swimming pool. Your assessment reveals that he is apneic and pulseless. The cardiac monitor reveals ventricular fibrillation. What precautions should be taken when using a defibrillator near water?

Putting It All Together

If the patient has monomorphic VT (and the patient's symptoms are due to the tachycardia):
- CPR and defibrillation are used if the patient is pulseless.
- Stable but symptomatic patients are treated with O_2, IV access, and ventricular antiarrhythmics (such as amiodarone) to suppress the rhythm.
- Unstable patients (usually a sustained heart rate of 150 beats/min or more) are treated with O_2, IV access, and sedation (if awake and time permits) followed by synchronized cardioversion.

   In all cases, an aggressive search must be made for the cause of the VT.

Putting It All Together

When administering procainamide, monitor the ECG closely for increasing PR intervals, increasing QT intervals (may precipitate Torsades de Pointes), widening of the QRS complex, and heart block.

Putting It All Together

- Sinus bradycardia
- Junctional rhythm
- Idioventricular (ventricular escape) rhythm
- AV conduction defects

Putting It All Together

Lead V_1
- Right side of sternum, fourth intercostal space

Lead V_2
- Left side of sternum, fourth intercostal space

Lead V_3
- Midway between V_2 and V_4

Lead V_4
- Left midclavicular line, fifth intercostal space

Lead V_5
- Left anterior axillary line at same level as V_4

Lead V_6
- Left midaxillary line at same level as V_4

Putting It All Together

The initial dosage should be 5 mcg/min delivered through an infusion pump capable of exact and constant delivery of the drug. Subsequent titration must be adjusted to the clinical situation, with dose increments becoming more cautious as partial response is seen. Initial titration should be in 5 mcg/min increments, with increases every 3 to 5 minutes until some response is noted. If no response is seen at 20 mcg/min, increments of 10 and later 20 mcg/min can be used. Once a partial blood pressure response is observed, the dose increase should be reduced and the interval between increments should be lengthened.

Putting It All Together

This patient is unstable (chest discomfort, altered level of consciousness, hypotension, difficulty breathing). Consider sedation, perform synchronized cardioversion with 50 J, and reassess the patient.

Putting It All Together

Because water conducts electricity, current can arc from one paddle or pad to the other if the patient's chest is wet, resulting in the delivery of less energy to the heart.

   If the patient and rescuer are in contact with water on the ground surface, it is possible that the rescuer may receive a shock or minor burn. This shock is typically not strong enough to seriously harm the rescuer, but may be uncomfortable.

   Before defibrillation, quickly dry the patient's chest and attempt to move the patient to a dry surface.

   Use cervical spine precautions if traumatic injury is suspected before moving the patient.

Putting It All Together

- Perform a primary survey (ABCs, O_2, IV, monitor)
- Assess vital signs, oxygen saturation
- Obtain SAMPLE history; assess patient's degree of discomfort
- Obtain 12-lead ECG, begin reperfusion checklist
- Evaluate 12-lead ECG and categorize the patient into one of three groups (ST-segment elevation, ST-segment depression, nondiagnostic/normal ECG)
- After making sure there are no contraindications, give 162 to 324 mg of baby aspirin
- After making sure the patient has not used Viagra, Cialis, or a similar medication in the past 24 to 48 hours, give nitroglycerin SL or spray and repeat every 5 minutes as needed to a maximum of 3 doses. Assess the patient's BP and pain 5 minutes after each dose. Prepare to give morphine IV if indicated.
- Get baseline cardiac biomarker levels, electrolytes, coagulation studies, chest x-ray
- Complete a reperfusion checklist, evaluate initial interventions, pain management

Putting It All Together

A 74-year-old man is complaining of weakness. He is pale, diaphoretic, and anxious. The cardiac monitor displays a second-degree AV block, type I, at 44 to 50 beats/min. The patient's blood pressure is 62/40, respiratory rate 16. Breath sounds are clear.

How will you manage this patient?

Putting It All Together

Briefly describe the initial management of a stable patient with polymorphic ventricular tachycardia and a normal QT interval.

Putting It All Together

Why is pain relief important in the management of the patient experiencing an acute coronary syndrome?

Putting It All Together

Describe how magnesium sulfate should be administered to a patient with a pulse.

Putting It All Together

What medications are recommended in the initial management of stable patients with a regular, wide-QRS tachycardia?

Putting It All Together

This rhythm strip is from an 83-year-old man complaining of weakness. He denies chest discomfort. Blood pressure is 62/40. Identify the rhythm (lead II) and describe your initial management of this patient.

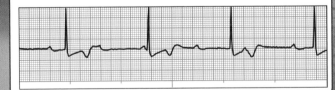

Putting It All Together

A 65-year-old woman is complaining of difficulty breathing. She is awake, anxious, and laboring to breathe. Examination reveals a blood pressure of 166/94, an irregular pulse rate of 90 to 120 beats/min, and a respiratory rate of 32. The skin is cool and moist. Auscultation of the chest reveals bilateral crackles. Pitting edema of the ankles is noted. The cardiac monitor shows atrial fibrillation. The patient has a history of hypertension for which she takes an antihypertensive medication.

How will you manage this patient?

Putting It All Together

This rhythm strip is from an unresponsive, apneic, and pulseless 20-year-old woman, the victim of a tricyclic antidepressant overdose. According to the roommate, she was awake (but groggy) 10 minutes ago. Identify the rhythm (lead I) and describe your initial management of this patient.

Putting It All Together

If the rhythm is polymorphic VT, it is important to determine if the patient's QT interval just before the tachycardia is normal or prolonged (if this information is available). If the QT interval is normal (that means the rhythm is polymorphic VT), the rhythm is sustained, and the patient is symptomatic due to the tachycardia:
- Treat ischemia if present.
- Correct electrolyte abnormalities.
- If the patient is stable, amiodarone may be effective. If the patient is unstable, proceed with defibrillation as for VF.

Putting It All Together

Mnemonic: "*A*ll *P*uppy *D*ogs *E*at"
Primary ABCD survey
Secondary ABCD survey (O$_2$, IV, monitor)
- *A*tropine 0.5 mg IV. May repeat every 3 to 5 minutes to a total dosage of 3 mg.
- *P*acing (transcutaneous). Pacing should not be delayed while waiting for IV access or for atropine to take effect.
- *D*opamine infusion 2 to 10 mcg/kg/min
- *E*pinephrine infusion 2 to 10 mcg/min

Putting It All Together

Magnesium sulfate is recommended for TdP (polymorphic VT with a prolonged QT interval with or without cardiac arrest). Some studies have shown that magnesium is also effective for atrial fibrillation with a rapid ventricular response. If the patient has a pulse, magnesium sulfate is given IV in a dose of 1 to 2 g diluted in D$_5$W over 5 to 60 minutes. If the patient is stable, infuse the drug slowly. If the patient is unstable, the drug can be given more rapidly.

Putting It All Together

Pain relief is a priority in the management of the patient experiencing an acute coronary syndrome because it
- Decreases anxiety and pain
- May decrease blood pressure and heart rate (reducing cardiac workload)
- Decreases myocardial oxygen demand
- Decreases the risk of dysrhythmias.

Putting It All Together

The rhythm shown is a complete AV block with ST-segment depression and inverted T waves.
Mnemonic: "*A*ll *P*uppy *D*ogs *E*at"
ABCs, O$_2$, IV, monitor
- *A*tropine 0.5 mg IV. May repeat every 3 to 5 minutes to a total dose of 3 mg.
- *P*acing (transcutaneous). Pacing should not be delayed while waiting for IV access or for atropine to take effect.
- *D*opamine infusion 2 to 10 mcg/kg/min.
- *E*pinephrine infusion 2 to 10 mcg/min.

Putting It All Together

The medications recommended in the initial management of stable patients with a regular, wide-QRS tachycardia are adenosine or amiodarone. Adenosine is given if the rhythm on the cardiac monitor is likely to be SVT with aberrant conduction. If the tachycardia is most likely ventricular tachycardia, amiodarone is the first drug that is recommended. Procainamide and sotalol are acceptable alternative choices. Amiodarone, procainamide, and sotalol are antiarrhythmics that have complex mechanisms of action. They are used for both atrial and ventricular dysrhythmias.

Putting It All Together

The rhythm shown is P-wave asystole. Begin CPR. Without interrupting CPR, start IV/IO. During CPR, give vasopressor: epinephrine 1 mg every 3 to 5 min or vasopressin 40 U × 1 in place of first or second epinephrine dose. Consider atropine 1 mg IV/IO repeated every 3 to 5 minutes to a maximum dose of 3 mg. Consider overdose-specific therapy, such as sodium bicarbonate per physician's order.

Putting It All Together

This patient is experiencing acute pulmonary edema. First-line treatment measures should include the following:
- If feasible, sit the patient up with the legs dependent
- Administer oxygen (be prepared to intubate if necessary)
- Establish IV access
- Administer sublingual nitroglycerin
- Administer furosemide 0.5 to 1.0 mg/kg
- Consider morphine administration

Putting It All Together

What situations/conditions can mimic ventricular fibrillation on the cardiac monitor?

Putting It All Together

The memory aid "PATCH-4-MD" may be used to recall possible treatable causes of cardiac emergencies. Explain the meaning of each of these letters.

Putting It All Together

This rhythm strip is from a 75-year-old man complaining of chest pain that has been present for 20 minutes. He rates his pain an 8 on a scale of 0 to 10. His blood pressure is 172/98. Identify the rhythm (lead II) and describe your initial management of this patient.

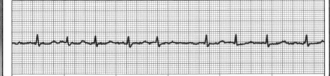

Putting It All Together

Name four advantages of endotracheal intubation.

Putting It All Together

How would you differentiate a junctional escape rhythm at 40 beats/min from a ventricular escape rhythm at the same rate?

Putting It All Together

A 66-year-old woman is found unresponsive, pulseless, and apneic. Emergency equipment and trained personnel are immediately available for assistance. Describe your initial interventions for this patient.

Putting It All Together

Briefly describe the initial management of a stable patient with polymorphic ventricular tachycardia and a prolonged QT interval.

Putting It All Together

This rhythm strip is from a 52-year-old man found unresponsive, apneic, and pulseless. Identify the rhythm (lead II) and describe your initial management of this patient.

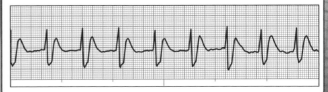

Putting It All Together

Pulmonary embolism
Acidosis
Tension pneumothorax
Cardiac tamponade
Hypovolemia
Hypoxia
Heat/cold (hyperthermia/hypothermia)
Hypokalemia/hyperkalemia (and other electrolytes)
Myocardial infarction
Drug overdose/accidents

Putting It All Together

- CPR
- Patient movement
- Loose or disconnected electrode

Putting It All Together

- Isolates the airway
- Keeps the airway patent
- Reduces the risk of aspiration
- Ensures delivery of a high concentration of oxygen
- Permits suctioning of the trachea
- Provides a route for administration of some medications
- Ensures delivery of a selected tidal volume to maintain lung inflation

Putting It All Together

The rhythm shown is atrial fibrillation with a ventricular response of 65 to 103/min.
   ABCs, O_2, IV, monitor
- Vital signs, pulse oximeter, blood pressure monitor
- SAMPLE history, assess discomfort (0 to 10 scale)
- Obtain 12-lead ECG
- Begin reperfusion checklist
- Give aspirin, nitroglycerin, morphine as indicated (if no contraindications)
   Evaluate 12-lead ECG (and categorize accordingly)
- Complete reperfusion checklist
- Get baseline cardiac biomarker levels, electrolytes, coagulation studies, chest x-ray
- Evaluate initial interventions, pain management

Putting It All Together

Verify that the scene is safe. Confirm that the patient is apneic and pulseless. If there is no pulse, and you witnessed the patient's collapse, perform CPR until a cardiac monitor/defibrillator is available. If there is no pulse and you did not witness the arrest, perform CPR for about 2 minutes and then analyze the patient's heart rhythm. If the monitor reveals a shockable rhythm (VT or VF), deliver one shock. After delivery of the shock, immediately resume CPR (or if the monitor reveals a nonshockable rhythm such as asystole or pulseless electrical activity), starting with chest compressions. Perform 5 cycles of CPR (about 2 minutes). Without interrupting CPR, start an IV/IO. During CPR, give a vasopressor (epinephrine or vasopressin). Assess the ECG rhythm and continue treatment in accordance with the appropriate algorithm.

Putting It All Together

A junctional escape rhythm is supraventricular in origin, thus it will have a narrow-QRS complex (0.10 second or less). A ventricular escape rhythm is ventricular in origin, thus it will have a wide-QRS complex (0.11 second or more).

Putting It All Together

Verify that the scene is safe. Confirm that the patient is apneic and pulseless. Despite the presence of an accelerated idioventricular rhythm on the cardiac monitor, the patient is pulseless. This situation is termed pulseless electrical activity (PEA). Resume CPR for about 2 min. Without interrupting CPR, start an IV/IO. During CPR, give a vasopressor (epinephrine 1 mg every 3 to 5 minutes or vasopressin 40 U × 1 in place of first or second epinephrine dose). Consider the possible causes of the arrest (PATCH-4-MD).

Putting It All Together

If the rhythm is polymorphic VT, it is important to determine if the patient's QT interval just before the tachycardia is normal or prolonged (if this information is available). If the QT interval is prolonged (that means the rhythm is TdP), the rhythm is sustained, and the patient is symptomatic due to the tachycardia:
- Discontinue any medications that the patient may be taking that prolong the QT interval.
- Correct electrolyte abnormalities.
- If the patient is stable, give magnesium sulfate IV. If the patient is unstable, proceed with defibrillation as for VF.

Putting It All Together

An Esophageal-Tracheal Combitube has been inserted. How should you confirm proper placement of the tube?

Putting It All Together

Name four disadvantages for using a simple face mask for oxygen delivery.

Putting It All Together

A 43-year-old woman is complaining of palpitations. She is alert and oriented × 4, blood pressure 168/96. Breath sounds are clear. She has a history of SVT and states that she cannot tolerate adenosine. Identify the rhythm and describe your initial management of this patient.

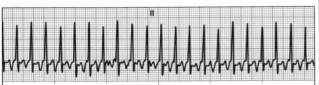

Putting It All Together

Why should the serum glucose level be determined during the initial management of a possible stroke patient?

Putting It All Together

This rhythm strip is from a 72-year-old man who is anxious and complaining of palpitations. Blood pressure is 110/64, pulse 190, and respirations 16. The patient denies chest pain. Breath sounds are clear. Identify the rhythm and describe your initial management of this patient.

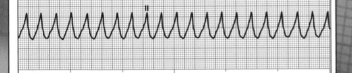

Putting It All Together

Name six life-threatening injuries that must be identified and treated in the primary survey.

Putting It All Together

An 80-year-old man has experienced a cardiac arrest. The cardiac monitor displays ventricular fibrillation. You have exposed the patient's chest and are applying combination pads to the patient's chest when you note that the patient has a permanent pacemaker in place. What distance from the pacemaker generator should the defibrillator pads be placed?

Putting It All Together

Identify the rhythm (lead II).

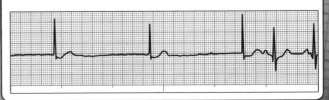

Putting It All Together

- Can only be used in a spontaneously breathing patient
- Not tolerated well in severely dyspneic patients
- Can be uncomfortable
- Difficult to hear the patient speaking when the device is in place
- Must be removed at meals
- Requires a tight face seal to prevent leakage of oxygen
- Oxygen flow rates of more than 10 L/min do not enhance delivered oxygen concentration

Putting It All Together

Fatal complications with the Combitube may occur if the position of the tube in the esophagus or the trachea is not correctly identified. After placement of the Combitube, use auscultation and inspection of chest rise as the primary methods of determining tube placement. These primary methods of determining tube placement must be supplemented with secondary confirmation with an exhaled CO_2 or esophageal detector device.

Putting It All Together

The serum glucose level should be determined during the initial management of a possible stroke patient because hypoglycemia can mimic the signs and symptoms of a stroke. The glucose test is performed to rule out hypoglycemia before proceeding with stroke treatment.

Putting It All Together

The rhythm is a narrow-QRS tachycardia with a ventricular response of about 214/min. Based on the information provided, the patient appears stable. Assess ABCs, administer O_2, start an IV, apply a monitor (already done), and obtain a 12-lead ECG. Attempt a vagal maneuver (if no contraindications). If unsuccessful, adenosine is usually given next but will be avoided because of the patient's intolerance to it. Consider a calcium channel blocker (verapamil, diltiazem) or a beta-blocker.

Putting It All Together

Life-threatening injuries that must be identified and treated in the primary survey include the following:
- Airway obstruction
- Open pneumothorax
- Tension pneumothorax
- Massive hemothorax
- Flail chest
- Cardiac tamponade

Putting It All Together

The cardiac monitor shows monomorphic ventricular tachycardia. Based on the information presented, the patient appears to be stable. The drug of choice for a stable patient in monomorphic VT is amiodarone. Because the patient has a pulse, give amiodarone 150 mg IV over 10 min. Repeat prn to a max dose of 2.2 g/24 hr. Alternative drugs include procainamide and sotalol.

Putting It All Together

Junctional bradycardia to sinus rhythm
- Ventricular rhythm: Regular (junctional beats); unable to determine (sinus beats)
- Ventricular rate: 30/min (junctional beats); unable to determine (sinus beats)
- Atrial rhythm: None (junctional beats); unable to determine (sinus beats)
- Atrial rate: None (junctional beats) to 75/min (sinus beats)
- PRI: None (junctional beats) to 0.18 (sinus beats)
- QRS: 0.04 second (junctional beats) to 0.08 (sinus beats)

Putting It All Together

Place defibrillator paddles or combination pads at least 1 inch (2.5 cm) from the pulse generator (bulge under the patient's skin). If the device is located in the patient's left pectoral area, standard sternum-apex paddle/pad placement for defibrillation is acceptable. If the device is located in the right pectoral area, anterior-posterior paddle/pad placement can be used.

Putting It All Together

The cardiac monitor shows a wide-QRS bradycardia at a rate of about 40. The patient has an altered mental status and his blood pressure is 50/P. A transcutaneous pacemaker is immediately available. What rate and output (mA) settings will you use for the pacemaker?

Putting It All Together

List three contraindications for sotalol use.

Putting It All Together

This rhythm strip is from a 62-year-old man complaining of palpitations. A synchronized shock was delivered, resulting in the following rhythm. Identify the rhythm (lead II).

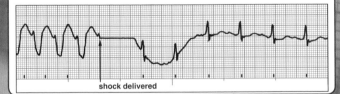

shock delivered

Putting It All Together

A 44-year-old woman is complaining of chest and left jaw pain, which she rates a 7 on a scale of 0 to 10. Blood pressure is 164/90, respirations are 18, and lung sounds are clear. Identify the rhythm and describe your initial management of this patient.

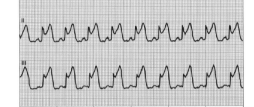

Putting It All Together

This rhythm strip is from an asymptomatic 72-year-old man. Identify the rhythm.

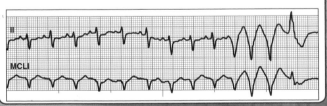

Putting It All Together

Name three preexisting conditions that can place an older adult at increased risk for stroke.

Putting It All Together

When intubating with a curved blade, where should the tip of the blade be positioned?

Putting It All Together

The following rhythm is observed on the cardiac monitor after administration of 6 mg adenosine IV. Identify the rhythm (lead II).

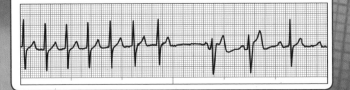

Putting It All Together

- Bronchial asthma
- Sinus bradycardia
- Second- and third-degree AV block (unless a functioning pacemaker is present)
- Congenital or acquired long QT syndromes
- Cardiogenic shock
- Uncontrolled CHF
- Previous evidence of hypersensitivity to sotalol

Putting It All Together

Initial transcutaneous pacemaker settings:
- Rate: start between 60 and 80 beats/min
- Output: start at minimum energy setting; gradually increase until capture; rate of increasing energy will depend on the patient's stability
- Assess electrical and mechanical capture

Putting It All Together

- Perform a primary and survey (ABCs, O₂, IV, monitor)
- Assess vital signs, oxygen saturation
- Obtain SAMPLE history; assess patient's degree of discomfort
- Obtain 12-lead ECG, begin reperfusion checklist
- Evaluate 12-lead ECG and categorize the patient into one of three groups (ST-segment elevation, ST-segment depression, nondiagnostic/normal ECG)
- After making sure there are no contraindications, give 162 to 324 mg of baby aspirin
- After making sure the patient has not used Viagra, Cialis, or a similar medication in the past 24 to 48 hours, give nitroglycerin SL or spray and repeat every 5 minutes as needed to a maximum of 3 doses. Assess the patient's BP and pain 5 minutes after each dose. Prepare to give morphine IV if indicated.
- Get baseline cardiac biomarker levels, electrolytes, coagulation studies, chest x-ray
- Complete reperfusion checklist, evaluate initial interventions, pain management

Putting It All Together

Monomorphic ventricular tachycardia to sinus rhythm with first-degree AV block
- Ventricular rhythm: Regular (sinus beats)
- Ventricular rate: 97/min (sinus beats)
- Atrial rhythm: Regular (sinus beats)
- Atrial rate: 97/min (sinus beats)
- PRI: 0.22 second (sinus beats)
- QRS: 0.10 second (sinus beats)

Putting It All Together

- Atherosclerosis
- Hypertension
- Immobility and/or limb paralysis
- Atrial dysrhythmias
- Congestive heart failure

Putting It All Together

Sinus tachycardia with a run of ventricular tachycardia
- Ventricular rhythm: Regular except for the event
- Ventricular rate: 135/min
- Atrial rhythm: Regular except for the event
- Atrial rate: 135/min
- PRI: 0.12 second
- QRS: 0.08 to 0.10 second

Putting It All Together

Conversion from narrow-QRS tachycardia to sinus rhythm
- Ventricular rhythm: Irregular
- Ventricular rate: 130/min (narrow-QRS tach) to 75/min (sinus beats)
- Atrial rhythm: Irregular
- Atrial rate: Unable to determine (narrow-QRS tach) to 75/min (sinus beats)
- PRI: 0.24 second (last sinus beat)
- QRS: : 0.08 second (last sinus beat)

Putting It All Together

The curved blade is inserted into the vallecula, the space or "pocket" between the base of the tongue and the epiglottis.

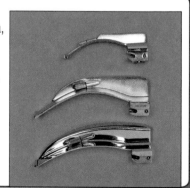

Putting It All Together

When intubating with a straight blade, where should the tip of the blade be positioned?

Putting It All Together

This rhythm strip is from a 59-year-old man who was driving to work on the freeway when his internal defibrillator discharged. He was asymptomatic at the time this ECG was obtained, a few minutes after the event. Identify the rhythm (lead II).

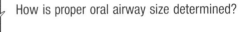

Putting It All Together

A 78-year-old woman is complaining of dizziness. She states that her symptoms began late yesterday evening and have become progressively worse. Her blood pressure is 78/40, respirations are 14, and lung sounds are clear. She denies chest pain and difficulty breathing. The cardiac monitor reveals the rhythm below. Oxygen is being administered and an IV has been established. Identify the rhythm (lead II) and describe the initial management of this patient.

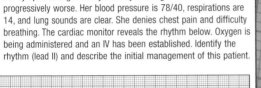

Putting It All Together

How is proper oral airway size determined?

Putting It All Together

Is condensation in the endotracheal tube a reliable indicator of proper tube position?

Putting It All Together

Explain the role of the resuscitation team member responsible for cardiopulmonary resuscitation (CPR).

Putting It All Together

Approximately 80% of strokes are of the _____ type; approximately 20% are of the _____ type.

Putting It All Together

Why is gastric distention a concern when delivering positive-pressure ventilation?

Putting It All Together

Atrial fibrillation
- Ventricular rhythm: Irregular
- Ventricular rate: 83 to 115/min
- Atrial rhythm: Unable to determine
- Atrial rate: Unable to determine
- PRI: Unable to determine
- QRS: 0.08 to 0.10 second

Putting It All Together

The tip of the straight blade is positioned under the epiglottis to expose the glottic opening.

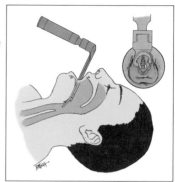

Putting It All Together

Proper airway size is determined by holding the device against the side of the patient's face and selecting an airway that extends from the corner of the mouth to the tip of the earlobe or the angle of the jaw.

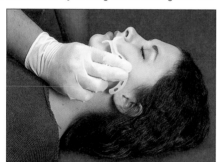

Putting It All Together

The monitor shows an idioventricular rhythm. Mnemonic: "*P*uppy *D*ogs *E*at"
Primary ABCD survey
Secondary ABCD survey (O$_2$, IV, monitor)
- *P*acing (transcutaneous)
- *D*opamine infusion 2 to 10 mcg/kg/min
- *E*pinephrine infusion 2 to 10 mcg/min

Putting It All Together

The Advanced Cardiac Life Support (ACLS) or Basic Life Support (BLS) team member responsible for CPR must know how to properly perform CPR and provide chest compressions of adequate rate, force, and depth in the correct location.

Putting It All Together

No. Multiple studies have confirmed that condensation in the endotracheal tube is not a reliable indicator of proper tube position. Further, chest rise and auscultation over the lungs and abdomen are also not reliable indicators of correct tube placement. To protect against unrecognized esophageal intubation, it is necessary to confirm tube position with an esophageal detector device, by monitoring exhaled CO$_2$, or by means of a chest x-ray.

Putting It All Together

Gastric distention is a complication of positive-pressure ventilation that can lead to regurgitation and subsequent aspiration. Gastric distention also restricts movement of the diaphragm, impeding ventilation.

Putting It All Together

Approximately 80% of strokes are of the <u>ischemic</u> type; approximately 20% are of the <u>hemorrhagic</u> type.

Putting It All Together

Name three causes of cardiac arrest other than atherosclerotic heart disease.

Putting It All Together

Hypotension may occur during acute myocardial infarction for several reasons. Name four possible causes of hypotension associated with a rate problem.

Putting It All Together

What is Wolff-Parkinson-White (WPW) syndrome?

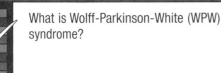

Putting It All Together

Name two signs of pericardial tamponade.

Putting It All Together

Explain the role of the resuscitation team member responsible for vascular access and medication administration.

Putting It All Together

Which of the following are contiguous leads?
- Lead II
- Lead V_4
- Lead aVF
- Lead III

Putting It All Together

Name at least five possible causes of sustained monomorphic ventricular tachycardia (VT).

Putting It All Together

You are instructed to administer amiodarone IV to a patient in atrial fibrillation. Describe how you will administer this medication.

Putting It All Together

Rate too fast:
- Sinus tachycardia
- Atrial fibrillation
- Atrial flutter
- PSVT
- Ventricular tachycardia

Rate too slow:
- Sinus bradycardia
- Second-degree AV block, type I
- Second-degree AV block, type II
- Third-degree AV block
- Pacemaker failure

Putting It All Together

- Trauma
- Hypoxia
- Drowning
- Electrocution
- Hypothermia
- Drug overdose
- Acid-base imbalance
- Electrolyte imbalance

Putting It All Together

Signs of pericardial tamponade may include the following:
- Hypotension
- Pulsus paradoxus
- Distended neck veins
- Muffled heart sounds
- Narrowing pulse pressure

Putting It All Together

WPW is a preexcitation syndrome in which an accessory pathway, called the Kent bundle, connects the atria directly to the ventricles, completely bypassing the normal conduction system. WPW is the most common preexcitation syndrome. It is more common in men than women. 60% to 70% of people with WPW have no associated heart disease. WPW is one of the most common causes of tachydysrhythmias in infants and children.

Putting It All Together

Leads II, III, and aVF are limb leads that look at the inferior wall of the left ventricle. Because these leads "see" the same part of the heart, they are considered contiguous leads. Lead V_4 is not contiguous. Remember: two leads are contiguous if they look at the same area of the heart or they are numerically consecutive chest leads. V_4 is a chest lead that looks at the anterior wall.

Putting It All Together

The Advanced Cardiac Life Support (ACLS) team member responsible for vascular access and medication administration should know the following:
- Site(s) of first choice for vascular access if no intravenous (IV) catheter is in place at the time of cardiac arrest.
- Procedure for performing intraosseous (IO) access in an adult.
- IV fluids of first choice in cardiac arrest.
- Importance of following each drug given in a cardiac arrest with a 20 mL IV fluid bolus and elevation of the extremity.
- Routes of administration and appropriate dosages for IV, IO, and endotracheal (ET) resuscitation medications.

Putting It All Together

Loading dose—150 mg IV bolus over 10 minutes (15 mg/min). May repeat every 10 minutes as needed. After conversion, follow with a 1 mg/min infusion for 6 hours and then a 0.5 mg/min maintenance infusion over 18 hours. Maximum cumulative dose is 2.2 g IV/24 hours.

Putting It All Together

Sustained monomorphic VT is often associated with underlying heart disease, particularly myocardial ischemia. It rarely occurs in patients without underlying heart disease. Common causes of VT include the following:
- Acute coronary syndromes
- Digitalis toxicity
- Cocaine abuse
- Acid-base imbalance
- Tricyclic antidepressant overdose
- Trauma (e.g., myocardial contusion, invasive cardiac procedures)
- Electrolyte imbalance (e.g., hypokalemia, hyperkalemia, hypomagnesemia)
- Cardiomyopathy
- Valvular heart disease
- Mitral valve prolapse

Putting It All Together

Name four signs and symptoms of hemodynamic instability that may occur as a result of a tachycardia.

Putting It All Together

A 75-year-old man is in cardiac arrest and CPR is in progress. Multiple attempts to establish a peripheral IV have been unsuccessful. What means of vascular access should be attempted next?

Putting It All Together

Why is hypotension secondary to pain management a complication that should be anticipated when treating right ventricular infarction (RVI)?

Putting It All Together

A 61-year-old man is complaining of weakness. His blood pressure is 72/48, respirations 16. Lung sounds are clear bilaterally. The cardiac monitor reveals the rhythm below. Identify the rhythm and describe your management of this patient.

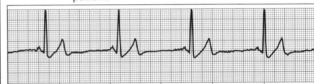

Putting It All Together

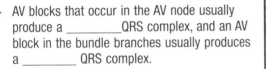

AV blocks that occur in the AV node usually produce a _____ QRS complex, and an AV block in the bundle branches usually produces a _____ QRS complex.

Putting It All Together

A patient with chest discomfort and ST-segment elevation is observed in leads II, III, and aVF. You have decided to obtain a right-sided 12-lead ECG. Where should the leads be placed?

Putting It All Together

Explain the role of the resuscitation team member responsible for ECG monitoring and defibrillation.

Putting It All Together

Complete the following table regarding nodal and infranodal AV blocks.

	Nodal block	Infranodal block
Coronary artery supply		
QRS width		
Patient stability		
Atropine response		
Cause		
Escape pacer		

Putting It All Together

If peripheral IV attempts are unsuccessful, intraosseous access should be attempted before trying a central line.

Putting It All Together

Examples of signs and symptoms of hemodynamic instability related to a tachycardia include the following:
- Altered mental status
- Shock
- Chest pain/discomfort
- Hypotension
- Shortness of breath
- Pulmonary congestion

Putting It All Together

The monitor shows a sinus bradycardia with ST-segment depression. Mnemonic: "*A*ll *P*uppy *D*ogs *E*at"
Primary ABCD survey
Secondary ABCD survey (O_2, IV, monitor)
- *A*tropine 0.5 mg IV. May repeat every 3 to 5 minutes to a total dosage of 3 mg.
- *P*acing (transcutaneous). Pacing should not be delayed while waiting for IV access or for atropine to take effect.
- *D*opamine infusion 2 to 10 mcg/kg/min
- *E*pinephrine infusion 2 to 10 mcg/min

Putting It All Together

In the setting of RVI, the infarction can reduce the output of the right ventricle, with a subsequent reduction in left ventricular filling. If such a decrease in preload does occur, it could potentially decrease left ventricular output as well. Morphine and nitroglycerin are vasodilators, and thus they reduce preload. This reduction in preload, although usually beneficial, can be undesirable in the setting of RVI and may cause profound hypotension. Therefore you must be cautious when administering nitroglycerin and morphine to patients experiencing RVI.

Putting It All Together

To view the right ventricle, right chest leads are used. Placement of right chest leads is identical to placement of the standard chest leads except on the right side of the chest. If time does not permit the acquisition of all six right-sided chest leads, the lead of choice is V_4R.

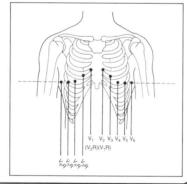

V_1 V_2 V_3 V_4 V_5 V_6
$(V_2R)(V_1R)$

Putting It All Together

AV blocks that occur in the AV node usually produce a <u>narrow</u> QRS complex (just as a junctional rhythm does), and an AV block in the bundle branches usually produces a <u>wide</u> QRS complex (just as a ventricular rhythm does). Although this rule is not absolute, it is another useful clue in determining the site of an AV block.

Putting It All Together

	Nodal block	Infranodal block
Coronary artery supply	*Right coronary artery*	*Left coronary artery*
QRS width	*Usually narrow*	*Usually wide*
Patient stability	*Generally stable*	*Often unstable*
Atropine response	*Usually improves*	*Often does not respond; may worsen*
Cause	*Usually increased parasympathetic tone*	*Usually serious tissue injury*
Escape pacer	*Junctional, usually reliable*	*Ventricular, often unreliable*

Putting It All Together

The Advanced Cardiac Life Support (ACLS) team member responsible for ECG monitoring and defibrillation should know the following:
- How to operate an automated external defibrillator (AED) and a manual defibrillator.
- The difference between defibrillation and synchronized cardioversion, and the indications for and potential complications of, these electrical procedures.
- The proper placement of hand-held defibrillator paddles and combination adhesive pads.
- The safety precautions that must be considered when performing electrical therapy.
- The indications for and possible complications of transcutaneous pacing.
- How to problem-solve equipment failure.

Putting It All Together

Name three situations in which the value of pulse oximetry may be limited.

Putting It All Together

A 62-year-old woman has a sudden onset of garbled speech and difficulty with movement on her right side. She has a history of hypertension. It is recommended that the interval from the time the patient arrives to the time the patient is seen by a physician should not exceed 10 minutes. Name the interventions that should be performed within the first 10 minutes of the patient's arrival.

Putting It All Together

When should the primary survey be repeated?

Putting It All Together

When might the AV junction assume responsibility for pacing the heart?

Putting It All Together

A 61-year-old woman has experienced a cardiac arrest. The cardiac monitor reveals ventricular fibrillation. CPR is ongoing, and defibrillation attempts have been unsuccessful thus far. Epinephrine has been administered. You are instructed to administer lidocaine. Indicate the initial dose of this medication, the repeat dose, the recommended interval between doses, and the maximum total dose that may be administered.

Putting It All Together

Cardiac tamponade is one possible cause of pulseless electrical activity. When gathering a patient's history, what information might lead you to suspect cardiac tamponade?

Putting It All Together

This rhythm strip is from a 67-year-old woman complaining of dizziness and a "funny feeling" in her chest. She denies chest pain and she is not short of breath. Her blood pressure is 112/92, respirations 22, lung sounds are clear. The cardiac monitor reveals the rhythm below. Describe your management of this patient.

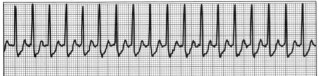

Putting It All Together

Identify the correct dose of epinephrine used in each of the following situations:
- Asystolic arrest—IV
- Symptomatic bradycardia—IV
- Ventricular fibrillation—endotracheal

Putting It All Together

- Assess ABCs, obtain vital signs
- Administer oxygen
- Obtain IV access
- Obtain blood samples (CBC, electrolytes, coagulation studies)
- Place patient on cardiac monitor
- Evaluate cardiac rhythm
- Obtain 12-lead ECG
- Check blood sugar and treat if indicated
- Alert stroke team: neurologist, radiologist, CT technician
- Perform general neurologic screening assessment

Putting It All Together

The value of pulse oximetry may be limited in the following situations:
- Anemia
- Hypothermia
- Cardiac arrest
- Peripheral edema
- Severe vascular disease
- Use of vasopressor therapy
- Carbon monoxide poisoning
- Hypotension (systolic blood pressure less than 50 mm Hg)

Putting It All Together

The AV junction may assume responsibility for pacing the heart if
- The SA node fails to discharge (e.g., sinus arrest)
- An impulse from the SA node is generated but blocked as it exits the SA node (e.g., SA block)
- The rate of discharge of the SA node is slower than that of the AV junction (e.g., sinus bradycardia or the slower phase of a sinus arrhythmia)
- An impulse from the SA node is generated and is conducted through the atria but is not conducted to the ventricles (e.g., AV block)

Putting It All Together

Repeat the primary survey
- With any sudden change in the patient's condition
- When interventions do not appear to be working
- When vital signs are unstable
- Before any procedures
- When a change in rhythm is observed on the cardiac monitor

Putting It All Together

History of the following:
- Trauma
- Recent fever
- Viral infection
- Previous cardiac surgery
- Acute myocardial infarction
- Chest pain
- Recent CPR
- Metastatic cancer

Putting It All Together

Lidocaine may be considered if amiodarone is not available. The initial dose of lidocaine is 1 to 1.5 mg/kg IV push. Repeat doses of 0.5 to 0.75 mg/kg IV push may be given at 5- to 10-minute intervals. The cumulative IV/IO bolus dose is 3 mg/kg. If there is a return of spontaneous circulation, consider a lidocaine infusion of 1 to 4 mg/min.

Putting It All Together

- Asystolic arrest—epinephrine 1 mg of 1:10,000 solution IV bolus
- Symptomatic bradycardia—epinephrine IV infusion, 2 to 10 mcg/min
- Ventricular fibrillation—epinephrine 2 to 2.5 mg (endotracheal dose); use 2 mg (2 mL) of 1:1000 solution; mix with 8 mL of normal saline (total volume = 10 mL) and administer down the ET tube

Putting It All Together

The ECG shows a narrow-QRS tachycardia with ST-segment depression. Based on the information provided, the patient is symptomatic, but stable. After assessing their ABCs, stable patients are given O₂ and an IV is started. A vagal maneuver can be attempted if there are no contraindications. If vagal maneuvers fail to convert a narrow-QRS tachycardia, adenosine is the first drug used to try to terminate the rhythm. Give adenosine 6 mg rapid IV bolus over 1 to 3 seconds.

If needed, administer adenosine 12 mg rapid IV bolus over 1 to 3 seconds after 1 to 2 minutes. May repeat 12 mg dose in 1 to 2 minutes if needed. Follow each dose immediately with 20 mL IV flush of normal saline. If a narrow-QRS tachycardia does not convert with adenosine (and the patient's condition remains stable), calcium channel blockers or beta-blockers may be used.

Putting It All Together

You are preparing to administer a lidocaine infusion. This medication is available in a premixed IV bag that contains 2 grams of lidocaine in 500 mL of IV solution. What is the concentration (milligram per milliliter) of this IV solution?

Putting It All Together

A 40-year-old man is complaining of dizziness. The cardiac monitor reveals a narrow-QRS tachycardia at 220 beats/min. Oxygen is being administered and an IV has been established. Blood pressure is 154/82. Vagal maneuvers were performed without success. You administered a 6 mg IV dose of adenosine and observed no change in the patient's cardiac rhythm; however, his BP is now 60/P and he does not respond to verbal or painful stimuli. The cardiac monitor remains unchanged. Describe your management of this patient.

Putting It All Together

An 81-year-old woman is complaining of chest pain that began 1 hour ago. She states that her pain began shortly after she noticed her "heart fluttering." She rates her pain a 4 on a scale of 0 to 10. Blood pressure is 82/50, respiratory rate is 26. Her skin is cool, pale, and moist. Lung sounds are clear. Oxygen is being administered and an IV has been established. The cardiac monitor reveals the following rhythm. Identify the rhythm and describe your management of this patient.

Putting It All Together

A 60-year-old man is complaining of dizziness and shortness of breath. His blood pressure is 70/38. Lung sounds reveal bibasilar crackles. His skin is cool, pale, and moist. Oxygen is being administered and an IV has been established. The cardiac monitor reveals the following rhythm. The patient appears hemodynamically unstable. Should cardioversion be performed at this time?

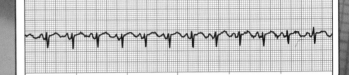

Putting It All Together

In the maintenance phase of a resuscitation effort, a spontaneous pulse has returned or the patient's vital signs have stabilized. Where should the efforts of the resuscitation team be focused during this phase?

Putting It All Together

A 65-year-old man has severe substernal chest pain that radiates to his left arm. He rates his pain a 9 on a scale of 1 to 10 and states that his symptoms began approximately 30 minutes ago. His blood pressure is 172/100. Oxygen is being administered and an IV has been established. A 12-lead ECG reveals ST-segment elevation in leads V_1, V_2, V_3, and V_4. Based on these ECG findings, what area(s) of the patient's heart is (are) affected? Describe the initial management of a patient experiencing an ST-segment elevation MI.

Putting It All Together

Name four possible causes of sinus tachycardia.

Putting It All Together

This rhythm strip is from a 62-year-old man complaining of dizziness. He denies chest pain. His blood pressure is 72/44.

Identify the rhythm (lead II) and describe your management of this patient.

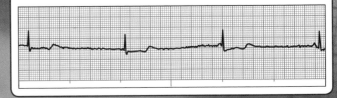

Putting It All Together

The patient is hemodynamically unstable. Perform synchronized cardioversion beginning with 50 J and increase to 100 J, 200 J, 300 J, and then 360 J (or equivalent biphasic energy) if the rhythm persists.

Putting It All Together

4 mg/mL

$$\frac{2\ g}{500\ mL} = \frac{2000\ mg}{500\ mL} = \frac{4\ mg}{1\ mL}$$

Putting It All Together

No. The rhythm on the cardiac monitor is a sinus tachycardia.

The purpose of synchronized cardioversion is to convert a dysrhythmia to one that is *sinus* in origin. This rhythm is already sinus in origin, although faster than normal. Cardioversion is not warranted in this situation. Look for and treat the underlying cause of the patient's sinus tachycardia.

Putting It All Together

The rhythm shown is monomorphic ventricular tachycardia.
The patient is hemodynamically unstable. Administer sedation and perform synchronized cardioversion beginning with 100 J (or equivalent biphasic energy). If the rhythm persists, cardiovert with 200, 300, and 360 J (or equivalent biphasic energy) as needed. Reassess the patient's response to each intervention.

Putting It All Together

ST-segment elevation in leads V_1, V_2, V_3, and V_4 suggests anteroseptal injury.
- Determine reperfusion strategy (fibrinolytics or percutaneous coronary intervention)
- Aspirin
- Beta-blockers
- Clopidogrel
- Heparin
- Angiotensin-Converting Enzyme (ACE) inhibitors (oral)
- Statins

Putting It All Together

Efforts of the resuscitation team should be focused on the following:
- Anticipating and preventing deterioration of the patient's condition
- Repeated assessment of the patient's ABCs
- Stabilizing vital signs
- Securing tubes and lines
- Troubleshooting any problem areas
- Preparing the patient for transport/transfer
- Accurately documenting the events during the resuscitation effort
- Drawing blood for laboratory tests and treating as needed based on results

Putting It All Together

The rhythm shown is a junctional bradycardia with ST-segment depression to sinus bradycardia with ST-segment depression and inverted T waves.
Mnemonic: "*A*ll *P*uppy *D*ogs *E*at"
Primary ABCD survey
Secondary ABCD survey (O_2, IV, monitor)
*A*tropine 0.5 mg IV. May repeat every 3 to 5 minutes to a total dose of 3 mg.
*P*acing (transcutaneous). Pacing should not be delayed while waiting for IV access or for atropine to take effect.
*D*opamine infusion 2 to 10 mcg/kg/min.
*E*pinephrine infusion 2 to 10 mcg/min.

Putting It All Together

Sinus tachycardia occurs as a normal response to the body's demand for increased oxygen due to fever, pain, anxiety, hypoxia, congestive heart failure, acute MI, infection, sympathetic stimulation, shock, hypovolemia, dehydration, exercise, and fright. Sinus tachycardia may also occur as the result of administration of medications such as epinephrine, atropine, dopamine, and dobutamine, or substances such as caffeine-containing beverages, nicotine, and cocaine.

Regardless of the outcome of the resuscitation effort or its length, the team leader is responsible for making sure that the resuscitation effort is critiqued by the team. What are the benefits of a critique, and what information should be reviewed during it?

You are preparing to administer a dopamine infusion. If you mixed 400 mg of dopamine in 250 mL of IV solution, what would the resulting concentration be?

Name three medications that may be used to sedate an awake patient before a procedure involving electrical therapy.

Tension pneumothorax is one possible cause of pulseless electrical activity (PEA). Name four findings that may be present on physical examination of the patient with a tension pneumothorax.

Putting It All Together

Putting It All Together

A critique of the resuscitation provides the following:
- An opportunity for education ("teachable moment")
- Feedback to hospital and prehospital personnel regarding the efforts of the team

Review the events of the resuscitation effort, including the following:
- Relevant patient history and events preceding the arrest
- Decisions made during the arrest and any variations from usual protocols

Discuss the elements of the resuscitation that went well, those areas that could be improved, and recommendations for future resuscitation efforts.

Putting It All Together

Putting It All Together

1600 mcg/mL

$$\frac{400 \text{ mg}}{250 \text{ mL}} = \frac{400,000 \text{ mcg}}{250 \text{ mL}} = \frac{1600 \text{ mcg}}{1 \text{ mL}}$$

Putting It All Together

Putting It All Together

Sedatives
- Diazepam (Valium)
- Midazolam (Versed)
- Etomidate
- Barbiturates
- Ketamine
- Methohexital (short-acting barbiturate)

Analgesics
- Fentanyl
- Morphine
- Meperidine

Putting It All Together

Putting It All Together

- Respiratory distress and/or arrest
- Hypotension
- Cyanosis
- Decreased or absent lung sounds on the affected side
- Tachypnea
- Tachycardia
- Mental status changes, including decreased alertness or responsiveness
- Hyperresonance of the chest wall on percussion
- Increasing resistance when providing positive-pressure ventilation
- Tracheal deviation (late finding)
- Jugular venous distention (may be absent if hypovolemia is present)
- Pulsus paradoxus

ILLUSTRATION CREDITS

Aehlert B: *ACLS study cards*, ed 2, St. Louis, 2004, Mosby.

Aehlert B: *ACLS study guide*, ed 3, St. Louis, 2007, Mosby.

Aehlert B: *ECG's made easy*, ed 3, St. Louis, 2006, Mosby.

Aehlert B: *ECG's made easy study cards*, St. Louis, 2004, Mosby.

Clochesy J, et al: *Critical care nursing*, ed 2, Philadelphia, 1996, WB Saunders.

Crawford M, et al: *Common sense approach to coronary care, revised*, ed 6, St. Louis, 1994, Mosby.

Drake R, et al: *Gray's anatomy for students*, New York, 2005, Churchill Livingstone.

Guyton A, et al: *Textbook of medical physiology*, ed 11, Philadelphia, 2006, WB Saunders.

Herlihy B: *The human body in health and illness*, ed 3, 2007, Mosby.

McSwain N, et al: *The basic EMT, revised,* ed 2, St. Louis, 2003, Mosby.

Sanders M: *Mosby's paramedic textbook, revised*, ed 3, St. Louis, 2007, Mosby.

Shade B, et al: *Mosby's EMT-Intermediate textbook for the 1999 National Standard Curriculum*, ed 3, St. Louis, 2007, Mosby.

Stoy W, et al: *Mosby's EMT-Basic textbook, revised*, ed 2, St. Louis, 2007, Mosby.

Stoy W, et al: *Mosby's EMT-Intermediate textbook, revised*, ed 2, St. Louis, 2007, Mosby.

Thibodeau G, et al: *Anatomy and physiology*, ed 6, St. Louis, 2007, Mosby.